Pathophysiology and Surgical Treatment of Unilateral Vocal Fold Paralysis

Eiji Yumoto

Pathophysiology and Surgical Treatment of Unilateral Vocal Fold Paralysis

Denervation and Reinnervation

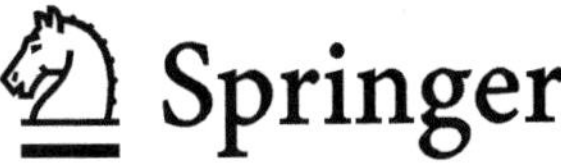 Springer

Eiji Yumoto
Department of Otlaryngology Head
    and Neck Surgery
Graduate School of Medical Sciences
    Kumamoto University
Kumamoto, Japan

ISBN 978-4-431-55353-3   ISBN 978-4-431-55354-0   (eBook)
DOI 10.1007/978-4-431-55354-0

Library of Congress Control Number: 2015937386

Springer Tokyo Heidelberg New York Dordrecht London

Printed on acid-free paper

Springer Japan KK is part of Springer Science+Business Media (www.springer.com)

Foreword

Many individuals have contributed to the art and science of phonosurgery over the last several decades. With pioneering achievements including those of Dr. Oskar Kleinsasser, Dr. Geza Jako, Dr. Harvey Tucker, Dr. John Conley, and then, of course, the great Dr. Minoru Hirano, and perhaps most notably Dr. Nobuhiko Isshiki. But it is on the shoulders of these greats that Dr. Eiji Yumoto takes the next step in creating a book that redefines and modernizes our thinking surrounding diagnostic and surgical laryngology.

This book provides a unique insight as to the value and the clinical potential for surgical techniques to address vocal fold paralysis focusing on laryngeal reinnervation and thyroplasty. These methods have evolved over time. Dr. Yumoto applies sound science to the techniques and provides a balanced and detailed description of the state of the art. This book stands apart due to its scientific rigor, clinically applicable information, and problem-focused approach. It is bound to contribute in an extremely meaningful way to the advancement of laryngology worldwide.

Chapter 1 provides a solid background to the anatomy and pathophysiology of vocal fold immobility. Included is a well-supported narrative describing the effects of recurrent laryngeal nerve injury and regeneration, the probable cause of vocal fold atrophy; synkinesis; glottis insufficiency; and vibratory deficits. The chapter is concluded with a rationale for appropriate therapeutic intervention.

Chapter 2 is dedicated to the evaluation and surgical treatment of vocal fold paralysis with a detailed analysis of prior published work and emphasizes the merits of reinnervation and highlights Dr. Yumoto's 15-year experience clinically managing this patient group.

Chapter 3 provides a basic science framework for the clinical finding identified with vocal fold denervation and reinnervation and includes data on the cellular effects of nerve–muscle pedicle flap implantation.

Chapter 4 discusses the diagnosis of paralytic dysphonia. The chapter includes the use and value of clinical voice measures, direct visual imaging, and the unique use of three-dimensional computer tomography and a new glottal configuration classification system. The chapter also contains valuable information on laryngeal electromyography.

Chapter 5 provides the details of the surgical technique of thyroarytenoid nerve–muscle pedicle flap reinnervation, which includes an analysis of patient outcomes, addressing phonatory and respiratory function as well as expected events and complications.

Chapter 6 summarizes the work and provides a framework for future directions for research and enhanced clinical care of the paralyzed vocal fold.

Certainly, I am very pleased to have the opportunity to preview the text and express my gratitude to the author for this contribution to our literature.

Madison, WI, USA   Timothy M. McCulloch

Preface

Vocal fold paralysis is a unique disease entity because clinical symptoms, degree of breathy dysphonia, and stroboscopic findings of vocal fold vibration differ from patient to patient. For example, some patients show over-adduction of the unaffected vocal fold over the midline during phonation while others do not even when a glottal gap exists. Prof. Nobuhiko Isshiki introduced laryngeal framework surgeries to surgically treat paralytic dysphonia. His idea was great in that the surgical methods were developed to modify position, mass, and tension of the vocal fold by changing the locational relation among thyroid, cricoid, and arytenoid cartilages without any intervention on vocal fold mucosa. Framework surgeries now have been popularized worldwide.

I started to work on these surgeries in the 1980s. Some patients recovered a very good voice, just like their own "pre-paralysis" voice, but unfortunately not all of them obtained a good voice although the postoperative voice definitely had improved compared with the preoperative voice. Based on the studies regarding vocal fold vibration with which I was involved for nearly 10 years from the latter half of the 1980s, I was convinced that, in addition to median location of the affected vocal fold, symmetrical mass, tension, and stiffness, thyroarytenoid (TA) muscle tonus is indispensable to recover the occurrence of the normal dynamic mucosal wave of the vocal fold.

Therefore, since I moved to Kumamoto University in 1998, my colleagues and I have been working to clarify denervation effects on the TA muscle and effects of the nerve-muscle pedicle (NMP) method on reinnervation of the TA muscle including muscle fibers, nerve fibers within the muscle, and neuromuscular junctions. The NMP method has been proven to reinnervate the denervated TA muscle and to be useful in recovering the "pre-paralysis" normal voice of each patient when combined with arytenoid adduction.

This book describes the pathophysiology and surgical treatment of unilateral vocal fold paralysis from the point of view of denervation and reinnervation.

I believe that we have arrived at a new horizon, having come from "static" adjustment by framework surgery alone to "dynamic" reconstruction by reinnervation combined with arytenoid adduction. Needless to say, as described in Chap. 6, much remains to be studied further.

Kumamoto, Japan   Eiji Yumoto, M.D.

Acknowledgments

It is my privilege to express my sincere gratitude to my mentors, Emeritus Prof. Naoaki Yanagihara and the late Associate Prof. Hiroshi Okamura, Ehime University, Japan, for their guidance and encouragement in laryngology. I also would like to express my sincere gratitude to Emeritus Prof. Nobuhiko Isshiki, Kyoto University, Japan, for his valuable advice.

I would like to acknowledge my great appreciation to the following colleagues who have spent a challenging time together carrying out basic animal experiments and clinical data analysis: Ryosei Minoda, Yasuhiro Samejima, Tetsuji Sanuki, Yoshihiko Kumai, Satoru Miyamaru, Takashi Aoyama, Yutaka Toya, Kohei Nishimoto, and Narihiro Kodama, Kumamoto University, Japan. All of them devoted themselves to the creation and refinement of this book.

Any inaccuracies in the text remain entirely my responsibility, but they have certainly been reduced by the very helpful and constructive comments on the manuscript by Edgardo S. Aberaldo, M.D., to whom special thanks are due. Finally and most importantly, I wish to thank my wife, Kyoko, for her patience and forbearance during the work on this book.

Contents

Chapter 1
Basic Knowledge of Vocal Fold Paralysis

Abstract Vocal fold paralysis is a pathological finding of motion impairment of varying degrees caused by nervous system disorders. In this chapter, the detailed anatomy of the laryngeal nerves and their varying anastomotic patterns within the larynx are described. Regeneration of nerve fibers after damage varies among patients. Significant misdirected regeneration occurs in some, whereas others show little synkinesis, which is a major cause of considerable inconsistencies of the vibratory pattern of the vocal folds among patients with unilateral vocal fold paralysis. Second, the effects of changes in the physical properties of the affected vocal fold on the production of the mucosal wave are summarized. Third, the factors that must be considered before surgical treatment of paralytic dysphonia are highlighted. Finally, reacquisition of the thyroarytenoid muscle tonus by reinnervation is important in recovering the preinjury voice with a dynamic mucosal wave.

Keywords Anastomosis of the laryngeal nerves • Misdirected reinnervation • Stiffness of the vocal fold • Synkinesis

1.1 What Is "Vocal Fold Paralysis"?

Vocal fold immobility is caused by various disorders, including damage of the recurrent laryngeal nerve (RLN), vagus nerve, or motor neurons and central nervous system, fixation or subluxation of the cricoarytenoid joint, adhesion of the posterior part of the vocal folds, tumor invasion into the intrinsic laryngeal muscle(s), and severe laryngeal edema. This book deals with vocal fold immobility and motion impairment due to nervous system disorders, with an emphasis on diagnosis of the pathophysiology of vocal fold paralysis and treatment aimed at reinnervation of the intrinsic laryngeal muscles.

"Recurrent laryngeal nerve paralysis (RLNP)" has been often used in clinical settings to indicate immobile vocal fold due to nerve damage. However, the vocal fold on the affected side is not always "fixed" and usually presents with slight movement during phonation and inhalation, although whether such motion is active or passive remains to be clarified. The position of the affected vocal fold ranges from median or paramedian to intermediate. The position sometimes shifts from an

Fig. 1.1 Combinations of injured nerves in vocal fold paralysis

1. Recurrent laryngeal nerve only

2. Recurrent laryngeal nerve and the external branch of the superior laryngeal nerve

3. Recurrent laryngeal nerve and the internal branch of the superior laryngeal nerve

4. Recurrent laryngeal nerve and the external and internal branches of the superior laryngeal nerve

5. Recurrent laryngeal nerve and lower cranial nerves (Glossopharyngeal, Vagal, Accessory, and Hypoglossal nerves)

intermediate to a median position as time elapses. As described later, electromyography (EMG) studies of most patients diagnosed with "RLNP" revealed the presence of laryngeal muscle activities, although they vary among individuals. The clinical diagnosis of "RLNP" includes varying degrees of nerve–muscle impairment: complete denervation of the superior and recurrent laryngeal nerves, resulting in total paralysis of the laryngeal muscles at one extreme and, as in most cases, partial denervation and reinnervation of the laryngeal muscles at the other extreme. Aberrant reinnervation may occur. Furthermore, the superior laryngeal nerve, including the internal and external branches and other lower cranial nerves, may be injured altogether (Fig. 1.1). Considering these issues, the term "vocal fold paralysis[1] (VFP)" rather than "RLNP" is used in this book.

1.2   Anastomotic Patterns of the RLN and Its Regeneration After Damage

The recurrent laryngeal nerve (RLN) is a branch of the vagal nerve and contains both motor and sensory fibers. After branching out from the vagal nerve, the RLN runs below the aortic arch posteriorly on the left side and below the subclavian artery posteriorly on the right side to proceed cranially along the tracheoesophageal groove; finally, it enters the larynx through the space between the thyroid and cricoid cartilages. Because the RLN runs a long distance due to its departure from the skull base to the larynx, the nerve can be damaged by various types of disease at different levels. Sensory fibers innervate the mucosa of the trachea and esophagus. A sensory branch called "Galen's branch" separates just before entering the larynx and makes an anastomosis with the internal branch of the superior laryngeal nerve (SLN) [1, 2]. Thus, the RLN after division of Galen's branch contains motor fibers. These fibers innervate the adductor muscles (thyroarytenoid muscle (TA), lateral cricoarytenoid muscle (LCA), arytenoid muscle (AR), and the abductor muscle (posterior cricoarytenoid muscle (PCA). Figure 1.2 shows schematically the

---

[1] "Paralysis" means loss or impairment of motor function due in part to a lesion of the neural or muscular mechanism (cited from Dorland's illustrated Medical Dictionary).

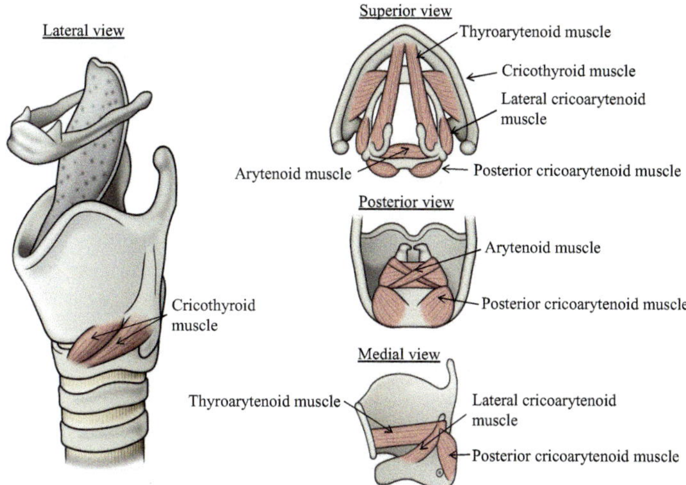

Fig. 1.2 Schematic illustration of the location of the intrinsic laryngeal muscles. The medial bundle of the thyroarytenoid muscle is called the "vocalis muscle"

arrangement of the intrinsic laryngeal muscles, including the cricothyroid muscle (CT), which is innervated by the SLN. The medial bundle of the thyroarytenoid muscle is called the "vocalis muscle" because of its significant role in the production and fine-tuning of the voice.

The SLN branches from the vagal nerve just below the inferior ganglion (i.e., the nodose ganglion), descends medially along the internal carotid artery, and then divides into internal and external branches. The internal branch (iSLN) contains mostly sensory fibers and enters the larynx through the thyrohyoid membrane or thyroid foramen (less often). The external branch (eSLN), which contains mainly motor fibers, descends along the connective tissue sheath containing the superior thyroid vessels and innervates the CT muscle.

The apparent position of the affected vocal fold varies among patients. As revealed by animal experiments [3–6] and clinical experiences [7–11], the laryngeal muscles almost always receive reinnervation after complete severance or even removal of a certain length of the RLN. Possible origins of regenerating nerve fibers have been reported not only from the RLN but also from branches of the vagal nerve to hypopharyngeal constrictor muscles, iSLN, eSLN, and autonomic nerves [2, 12–18]. Nasri et al. confirmed the presence of the motor nerve supply from eSLN to the TA muscle electromyographically in three of seven canine models [19]. Sanders et al. investigated the gross anatomy and interactions between SLN and RLN in human larynges [14]. They found connections between these nerves, with the exception of Galen's anastomosis: (1) the RLN combines with the SLN in the neural plexus at the AR muscle; (2) the AR branches of the bilateral RLNs anastomose with each other; (3) the eSLN passes from the CT muscle and has a connection with the TA muscle branch of the RLN; and (4) the PCA branch of the RLN interacts with the AR branch. They indicated that there are significant neural connections between the RLN and SLN and that limited cross-innervation is seen from side to side in the area of the AR muscle. However, some connections were variable among the larynges, suggesting that the regeneration pattern after RLN injury would be determined individually considering these variations.

Semon reported a paralyzed vocal fold positioned at the median or paramedian position at the onset of VFP that gradually changed in position laterally. He explained this shift by assuming that the nerve fibers supplying the PCA muscle are more sensitive to injury than are the nerve fibers to the adductor muscles [20]. However, a time-dependent shift in a paralyzed vocal fold from a median to an intermediate position is rarely observed in a clinical setting as reported by Faaborg-Anderson [21]. The Wagner–Grossman theory[2] has also been abandoned following recent experimental and clinical studies [6, 11, 23, 24].

Sanudo et al. scrutinized nerve connections in the human larynx and found four different anastomoses between the RLN and iSLN: (1) Galen's anastomosis; (2) arytenoid plexus, including connections between the dorsal branch of the iSLN and ventral branch of the RLN in the mucosa and the AR muscle and connections to the contralateral side; (3) cricoid anastomosis between the arytenoid plexus and RLN branch before entering the larynx; and (4) thyroarytenoid anastomosis between the descending branch of the iSLN and ascending branch of the RLN. Anastomosis between the eSLN and RLN appears as a connecting branch throughout the CT muscle [2]. The various prevalences of the anastomotic patterns of this complex suggest functional differences in the regeneration of the sensory and motor fibers among individual subjects. Maranillo et al. also reported that some of the LCA and TA muscles receive a nerve supply from the iSLN or eSLN in addition to the RLN [25]. These anastomotic patterns vary among individuals and between the sides. When a motor fiber is transected, adjacent fibers sprout, extend into the remaining Schwann sheath, and reach a muscle to reinnervate before it falls into degeneration [26]. When the RLN is injured, nerve fiber regeneration occurs through the above-mentioned anastomotic routes to supply motor fibers to each muscle. However, such reinnervation patterns differ among individuals. Regeneration is not limited to motor fibers but may also include autonomic systems. Thus, it seems there is no definite rule regarding what determines the position of the affected vocal fold.

Damrose et al. electrically stimulated the RLN when they performed arytenoid adduction on 15 patients and failed to detect any evoked potentials from the TA muscle. They concluded that little regeneration occurs through the RLN after its damage [27]. However, because surface electrodes on the skin were applied in 11 of 15 patients in their study, electrical activities of relatively small amplitude may have not been detected. It is generally accepted that the contraction strength and the timing of each laryngeal muscle influence the position of the "paralyzed" vocal fold. Another factor that may affect vocal fold position is the expiratory airflow. The

---

[2]The activities of the cricothyroid muscle are assumed to be responsible for the preponderance of the median position among paralyzed vocal fold positions [22].

expiratory airflow pushes the affected vocal fold upward and laterally when TA muscle contraction is insufficient.

Despite the accumulated evidence that the intrinsic laryngeal muscles receive a regenerated nerve supply in both animal models and patients, why physiological vocal fold movement fails to recover fully remains to be determined. Misdirected regeneration or synkinesis is considered to be the main cause [11, 16, 24, 28–37]. Many sprouting fibers grow from the central end of the nerve sheath after transection, and those that reach the myelin sheath on the peripheral side extend to make connections with target muscle fibers. Such growth of nerve fibers is very active, and their extension shows no target organ specificity [38]. The RLN innervates both adductor and abductor muscles, and fibers toward these muscles intermingle in the main nerve until it branches [26, 39–41]. Thus, the regenerated fibers have very little opportunity to reach and innervate the original target muscle. Further, a single nerve fiber may innervate both adductor and abductor muscle fibers (Fig. 1.3). The RLN contains not only motor fibers but also sensory and autonomic components [42], and regenerated fibers may connect with these non-motor fibers and vice versa. Second, only a few nerve fibers successfully reach the myelin sheath on the peripheral side, resulting in a decrease in the number of reinnervated muscle fibers [43]. Third, sufficient muscle contraction fails to recover even after reinnervation because laryngeal muscles degenerate during periods of denervation, accompanied by atrophic and fibrotic changes (Fig. 1.4) [44].

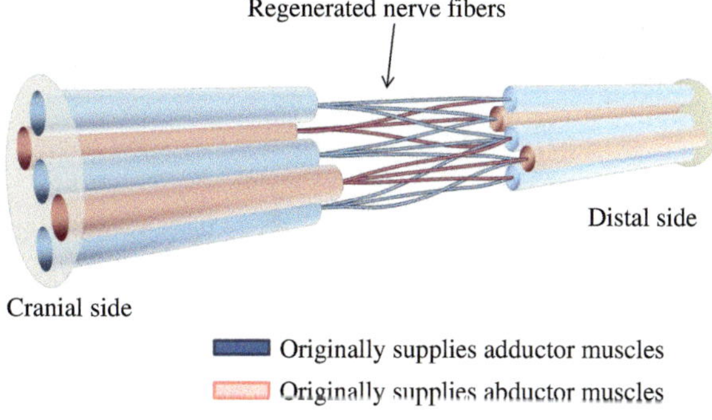

Fig. 1.3 Regenerated nerve fibers after denervation, showing possible misdirections. Regenerated fibers extend toward an original target muscle as well as its opponent muscle

Fig. 1.4 Possible causes of the failure of physiological vocal fold movement to recover after injury. Items *1–3* indicate factors related to misdirected regeneration of nerve fibers, and items *4* and *5* indicate those unrelated to misdirected regeneration

1. Nerve fibers innervate antagonistic muscle fibers. (ie abductor branch reaches adductor muscle fiber and vice versa)

2. A single nerve fiber innervates both adductor and abductor muscle fibers.

3. Nerve fibers regenerate into nerve sheaths of different nature. (ie motor fiber to sensory or autonomic fiber and vice versa)

4. Nerve fibers fewer than the cranial side reach the myelin sheath on the distal side.

5. Laryngeal muscles degeneration. (ie denervated muscles fail to recover sufficient muscle contraction even after reinervation)

1.3   Symptoms

Unilateral vocal fold paralysis (UVFP) causes breathy hoarseness of varying degrees from a subtle change to a nearly aphonic state and swallowing difficulties. When the affected vocal fold is located off the midline, expectoration of food residue, sputum, and saliva in the supraglottic space and pyriform sinus becomes less effective because of insufficient elevation of subglottic pressure during coughing [45, 46]. Furthermore, latent penetration into the trachea may occur due to diminished sensation of laryngeal mucosa [47–49]. Unless other lower cranial nerve injuries are involved, dysphagia is usually mild and resolves in 10–20 days after onset. On the other hand, breathy dysphonia interferes with verbal communication, resulting in difficulty in social activities and physical symptoms such as fatigue, exhaustion, or numbness of the body due to hyperventilation after conversation. These symptoms definitely reduce the quality of life in patients with UVFP [50–53].

The symptoms of bilateral vocal fold paralysis are different from those of UVFP and depend mainly on the fixed position and residual motility of the vocal folds. When the glottis is wide (i.e., the vocal folds are fixed at an intermediate position), patients complain of breathy dysphonia without respiratory distress. When the glottis is narrow (i.e., the vocal folds are fixed in a median or paramedian position), inspiratory dyspnea is the main concern, although the voice is not hoarse. When the vocal fold positions are paramedian with slight vocal fold movement, the patients remain asymptomatic. Those with bilateral vocal fold paralysis who visit the ear, nose, and throat clinic are often indicated for tracheostomy or surgery to widen the glottis for relief of exertional dyspnea.

1.4   Vocal Fold Vibration

Considerable inconsistencies regarding the vibratory pattern of the vocal fold among patients with UVFP exist. Stroboscopic examination reveals that the closed phase during a vibratory cycle becomes very short or even absent. A mucosal wave may be irregular among cycles or asymmetric between the vocal folds due to the differences in the mass, tension, and stiffness of the vocal folds. Furthermore, stroboscopic illumination may not show vibratory images of the vocal folds when the acoustic signal of the voice does not contain periodic signals, specifically when the patient's voice is extremely breathy. On aerodynamic examination, the maximum phonation time (MPT) decreases, the mean airflow rate (MFR) increases, and laryngeal efficiency such as the vocal efficiency index [54] is diminished. The auditory impression of the voice is characteristic in that breathiness is enhanced according to the GRBAS scale [55]. A normal vocal fold vibration is a result of vocal folds positioned midline, pliable vocal fold mucosa, and symmetrical physical properties such as shape, thickness, mass, stiffness, and tension. In patients with UVFP, in addition to the off-midline position of the vocal fold, lowered stiffness and tension, reduced thickness of the vocal fold, atrophic changes of the TA muscle, and synkinetic movement of the vocal fold on the affected side cause negative effects on vocal fold vibration.

1.4.1   Glottal Insufficiency

When normal vocal fold vibration begins in a soft attack mode, a slight prephonatory glottal gap exists; this closes following elapse of a few vibratory cycles [56]. However, the glottal gap remains even after several periods in patients with UVFP. Thus, glottal airflow is constantly leaked excessively through the glottis, which makes airflow turbulent rather than laminar, resulting in high-frequency noise (Fig. 1.5).

1.4.2   Atrophy of the Thyroarytenoid Muscle

Kobayashi et al. examined the effects of unilateral atrophy of the TA muscle on its vibratory mode in excised canine larynges [57]. The unilateral RLN was removed for a distance of 10 mm, and its proximal stump was sutured into the sternothyroid muscle to prevent reinnervation. The larynx was harvested 4 months after the procedure to allow the muscle to atrophy. Both vocal processes were sutured together to attain posterior glottal closure, and the larynx was fixed in a custom-made apparatus. The thyroid ala of the atrophied side was pressed medially to obtain sufficient glottal closure for steady phonation. Lateral and vertical displacements were measured simultaneously during phonation. Kobayashi et al. reported three main findings: (1) the vibration in the unilaterally atrophied larynges was periodical and symmetrical in phase, (2) the lateral amplitude was significantly greater than the vertical amplitude on both sides, and (3) the lateral and vertical amplitudes on the atrophied side were significantly greater than those on the normal side (Figs. 1.6 and 1.7) [57]. Thus, in the minimal prephonatory glottal gap, periodic vibration occurs in unilaterally atrophied larynges, and the amplitude is greater in the lateral and vertical directions than in the normal fold. The latter finding implies that phonosurgical procedures aimed at closure of the prephonatory glottal gap may have a

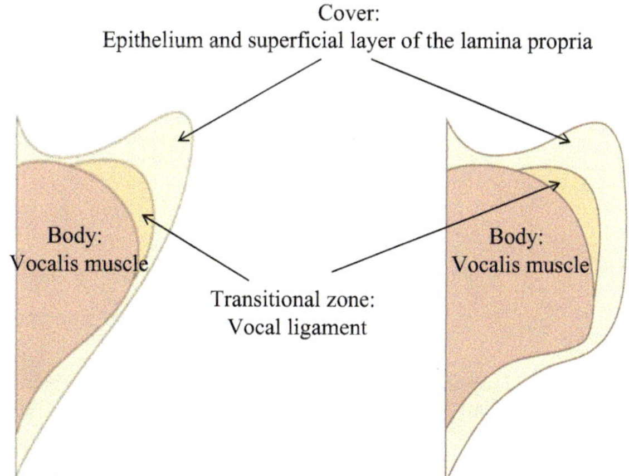

Fig. 1.5 Schematic illustration of the coronal section of the human vocal fold. *Left*: without contraction of the thyroarytenoid muscle; *Right*: with contraction of the thyroarytenoid muscle. Relative to actual thicknesses, the lamina propria is enlarged to facilitate understanding. Subsequent figures are drawn in a similar way

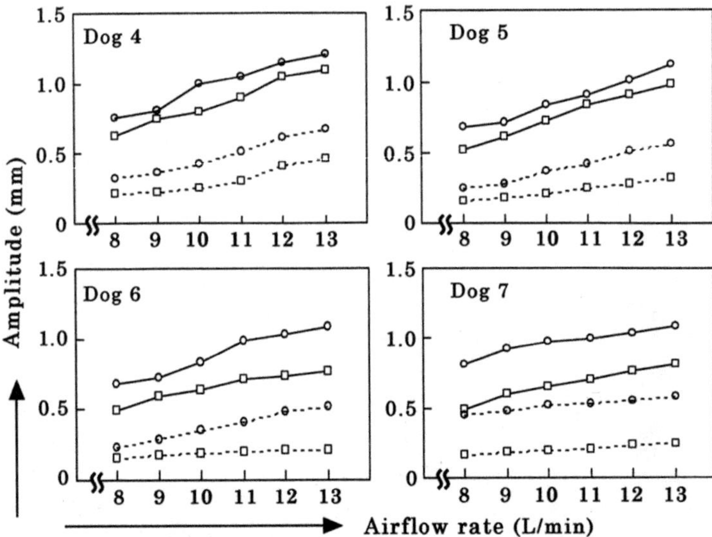

Fig. 1.6 Lateral and vertical amplitudes in the four unilaterally atrophied larynges. The horizontal axis represents the airflow rate (liters per minute), and the vertical axis represents lateral (*solid line*) and vertical (*dotted line*) amplitudes. Circles represent the amplitude on the atrophied side; squares represent the amplitude on the normal side (Citation: Ref. [57])

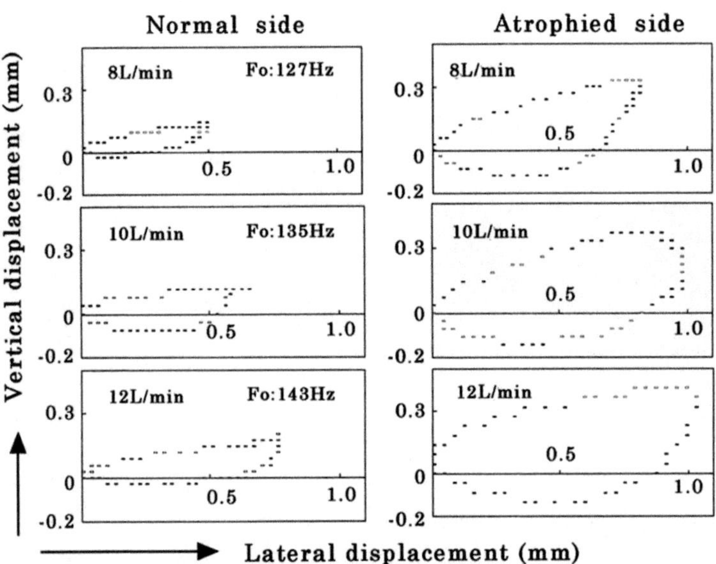

Fig. 1.7 Lissajous trajectories of the vocal fold in a representative case when the larynx was blown at three different airflow rates. The horizontal and vertical axes represent lateral and vertical displacements of the vocal fold in millimeters, respectively (Citation: Ref. [57])

beneficial effect on hoarseness in UVFP patients, although displacements of the vocal folds during vibration are not symmetrical.

1.4.3   Lowered Stiffness and Tension of the Vocal Fold

The human vocal fold comprises the muscle layer (medial part of the TA muscle, vocalis muscle), vocal ligament, and mucosa (which consists of a very thin epithelial layer and a loose superficial layer of the lamina propria) (Fig. 1.5, left). Mechanical properties vary depending on the degree of contraction of the vocalis muscle. The vocal ligament consists of deep and intermediate layers of the lamina propria. The former is composed of dense fibrous tissue and is tightly connected with the muscle layer. The latter contains elastic and collagen fibers and functions as a transitional zone from the muscle layer to the superficial layer. The mucosa is connected loosely with the vocal ligament and can be moved in a different manner from that of the muscle layer. Hirano reported that the vocal fold could be regarded as a double-structured vibrator consisting of a body comprising the vocalis muscle and vocal ligament and a cover consisting of the epithelium and loose superficial layer of the lamina propria. A mucosal wave observed during phonation is elicited primarily by the cover [58].

When the CT muscle contracts, the vocal fold is elongated and becomes thinner, resulting in the elevation of the vocal fold tension. Such changes in tension produce a higher-pitch voice. On the other hand, contraction of the TA muscle causes bulging of the medial–inferior surface of the vocal fold and elevation of stiffness of the body of the vocal fold. The author and his colleagues investigated the effect of TA muscle contraction on the shape of the subglottic vault using a canine model [59]. The subglottic vault surrounded by the lower surface of the vocal fold formed a concave shape in the absence of TA muscle contraction and became convex during TA muscle contraction. The cover becomes relatively less stiff—i.e., more pliable—resulting in the more vigorous occurrence of a mucosal wave. In the human larynx, the cover is much thinner than the canine; thus, during moderate contraction of the CT muscle, TA muscle contraction plays a greater role in adjusting the stiffness of the whole vocal fold. During strong CT contraction, the cover is stretched, and its tension increases, diminishing the influence of TA muscle activity in the overall stiffness of the vibrating part of the vocal fold [60–63]. Sercars et al. reported a case of UVFP producing a voice with higher activities of the CT muscle [64]. They inferred that the strong CT muscle contraction elevated the tension of the cover and minimized the imbalance of stiffness between the vocal folds. As a result of such laryngeal adjustment, airflow escape during phonation decreases, and the voice becomes high pitched. Such compensatory phonation is termed "paralytic falsetto."

Paralysis of the CT muscle produces asymmetry of vocal fold tension in the anterior–posterior direction. Based on animal studies, Tanabe et al. and Isshiki et al. found that, in such cases with a closed glottis, the vocal fold vibration is periodic with the vocal fold on the active side preceding the paralyzed side in the vibratory cycle, and the generated sound is not hoarse. With a wider glottal gap, glottal closure becomes irregular with less periodic vibration, and the voice is hoarse [65, 66]. Maunsell et al. reported similar results and theorized that a "coupling effect" occurs between the asymmetric vocal folds despite the presence of imbalance in tension, stiffness, and mass when disparities are insignificant [67]. They also reported that as airflow increases, the phase difference between the vocal folds decreases.

The author observed vocal fold vibration of the excised canine larynges from the tracheal side using a high-speed movie technique and found that the mucosal upheaval (MU), where the mucosal wave starts and propagates upward, appears between the anterior commissure and vocal process on the lower surface of the vocal fold when the vocal fold vibrates [68–71]. The pliability of the vocal fold mucosa was measured along the superior–inferior axis in the canine larynx. Pliability was defined as the maximal elevated distance in response to a constant focal negative pressure (−300 mmHg) applied through a 22-gauge needle with a flat tip (Fig. 1.8) [72]. After confirming contact of the needle tip with the mucosal surface under the operating microscope, the needle tip was slowly moved away using a micromanipulator. Thus, the mucosa was pulled off its original position by the needle tip until it was detached from the mucosa. These two critical moments when the mucosa and needle tip come into contact and become separated were carefully observed, and the distance between these two points was measured by the micromanipulator to an accuracy of 10 μm. It was revealed that the MU where the mucosal wave starts occurs around the point of minimal pliability [72]. Histological examination revealed that the MU occurred where the lamina propria became thinner and

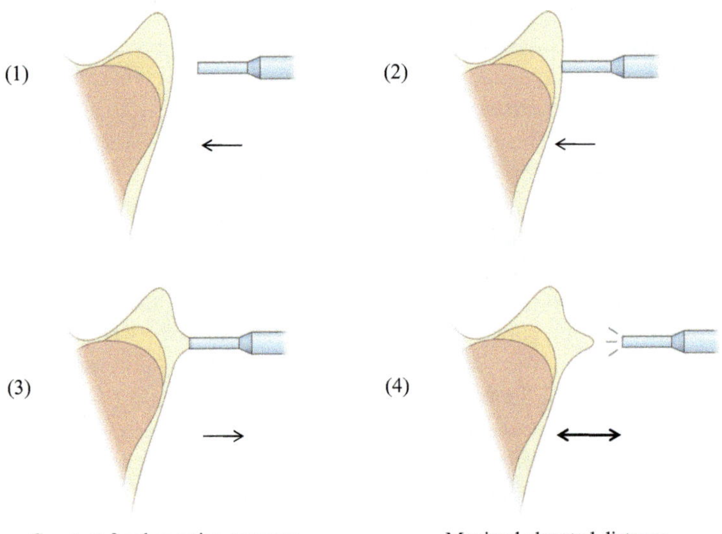

Fig. 1.8 Schematic representation of the method used to measure the pliability of the vocal fold mucosa (Modified from Refs. [63, 72])

where the muscle layer neared the epithelial layer. When the vocal fold is lengthened, the MU actually shifts medially to the area where the lamina propria becomes thicker and where the free edge of the vocal fold is closer [69, 70].

Conversely, contraction of the TA muscle caused the lower surface of the vocal fold to bulge medially and to narrow the subglottic vault surrounded by the bilateral MU. The MU moved to the tracheal side during TA muscle contraction compared with its initial position when the TA muscle is relaxed. Therefore, TA muscle contraction causes expansion of the vibrating area toward the tracheal side and contributes to the production of a more dynamic mucosal wave in the vertical direction (Fig. 1.9) [59, 63, 71]. Although the cover of the human vocal fold is thinner than that of the canine, observation of the lower surface of the vocal folds through a tracheostomy confirmed the presence of MU in humans and that the mucosal wave starts at this point and propagates upward [73, 74]. Insufficient activities of the TA muscle due to UVFP may impair the development of MU, and the mucosal wave is not generated dynamically. Therefore, the patient's voice becomes weak with little strength in addition to breathiness due to air escape through the glottis.

Sanders et al. proposed that the human TA muscle has two functionally different parts: the lateral part for vocal fold adduction and the medial part for phonation (vocalis muscle) [75]. The vocalis muscle is further divided into superior and inferior subcompartments (SCs): the superior SC is composed of numerous small fascicles where muscle fibers are loosely arranged and of different sizes, while the inferior SC has a single large muscle fascicle densely packed with muscle fibers

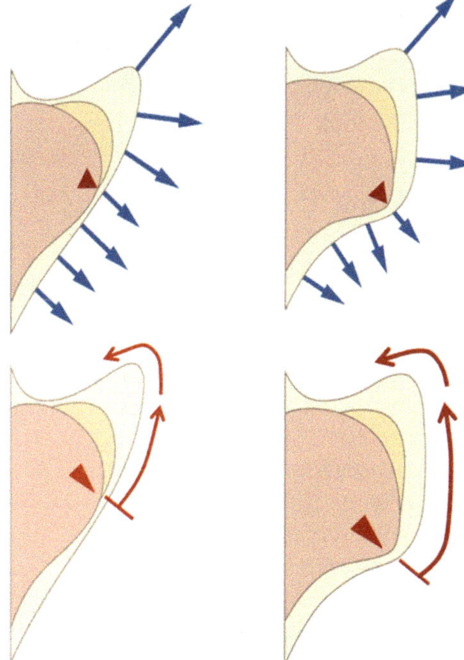

Fig. 1.9 Mucosal pliability (*upper*) and mucosal wave (*lower*) without TA muscle contraction (*left*) and with TA muscle contraction (*right*). When the TA muscle contracts, the lower surface of the vocal fold bulges medially and becomes thicker. The point of minimum pliability moves toward the tracheal side, and a more dynamic mucosal wave is elicited in the vertical direction. The length of *arrows* indicates the pliability of the mucosa, *red triangles* show the position of minimum pliability, and the *red arrows* indicate the area in which the mucosal wave occurs

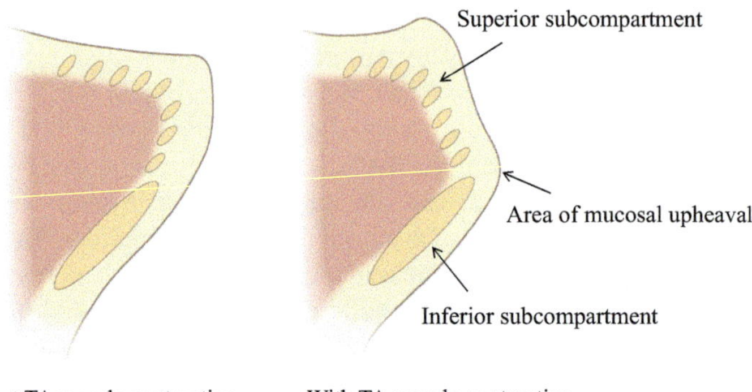

Fig. 1.10 Superior and inferior subcompartments of the vocalis muscle with (*right*) and without (*left*) thyroarytenoid muscle contraction (Modified from Ref. [77])

(Fig. 1.10). The superior SC seems to be a unique entity in the human vocal fold because the superior SC area is mostly composed of soft tissue in most animals. Sanders et al. also reported that muscle spindles in the TA muscle are concentrated in the superficial part of the superior SC of the vocalis muscle [76]. Based on these findings and the author's reports regarding the MU, it is likely that the MU occurs along the transitional area between the superior and inferior SCs of the vocalis muscle. Thus, the superior SC is likely to be involved in the mucosal wave, and the rich presence of muscle spindles in the superior SC may have a role in adjusting the development and progression of the mucosal wave. These reports are congruent with the author's observations that a superficial part of the TA is involved in the vibratory movement of the vocal fold [59].

1.5 What Should Be Done to Obtain a "Normal Voice"?

Many surgical methods, including type I thyroplasty, arytenoid adduction, intra-cordal injection, and combinations thereof, have been reported to treat breathy hoarseness due to UVFP. These methods aim at closure of the glottal gap and increasing the thickness of the affected vocal fold. Postoperative voices in most cases improve. However, they rarely return to the patient's own "normal" voice before the onset of UVFP. Based on what has been discussed thus far, several areas have not been addressed by conventional phonosurgeries, leaving an area for refinement of surgical techniques. As mentioned in Sect. 1.4, it is equally important to address the symmetry of the vocal fold mass, tension, stiffness, and mucosal pliability as to address medializing the paralyzed folds. Conventional surgical methods can achieve these items to a certain degree but cannot replace the role of the TA muscle in the adjustment of physical properties of the vocal fold, particularly tension of the cover and stiffness of the whole vocal fold.

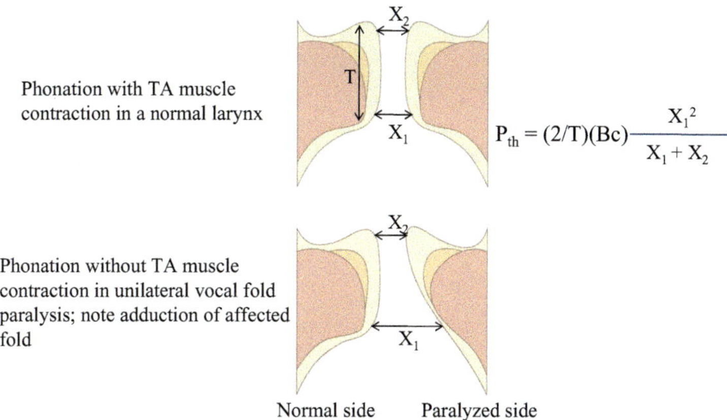

Fig. 1.11 The prephonatory glottal shape in the coronal section and minimum lung pressure required for the onset of the vocal fold oscillation (phonation threshold pressure (P_{th}))

The phonation threshold pressure (P_{th}), the minimum lung pressure required for the onset of vocal fold oscillation, can be determined using the following equation for a glottal shape, as shown in Fig. 1.11:

$$P_{th} = (2/T)(Bc)\left(X_1^2 / (X_1 + X_2)\right)$$

where T represents vocal fold thickness, B is a viscous damping coefficient in the tissue, c is the mucosal wave velocity, and X_1 and X_2 represent the distances between the vocal fold at the inferior and superior surfaces of the vocal fold, respectively, at the prephonatory phase [77]. P_{th} is regarded as an indicator of the ease of phonation. P_{th} increases as X_1 increases, indicating that the "ease of phonation" is reduced by a greater separation of the vocal fold at the bottom. Only TA muscle contraction can achieve a medial–inferior bulge of the vocal fold during phonation. Procedures of insertion of artificial materials (type I thyroplasty) and intracordal injection cannot always recover such vocal fold shape and stiffness and perform fine adjustments of the vocal fold during phonation. Therefore, reacquisition of the thyroarytenoid muscle contraction by reinnervation is considered essential for the successful recovery of a preparalysis normal voice with a dynamic mucosal wave.

1.6   Factors to Be Considered During Diagnosis

In addition to the presence of UVFP, the pathological situation of the affected fold and vocal fold vibration should be evaluated carefully. Videoendoscopy under stroboscopic illumination is one of the most useful methods of observing the larynx. However, the observation is from the oral side and with a single vision. Thus, three-dimensional (3D) configuration of the vocal fold is not fully assessed (Fig. 1.12).

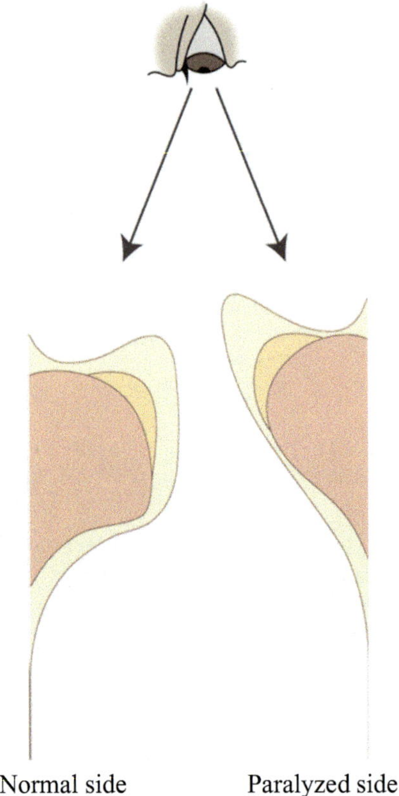

Fig. 1.12 Observation of the larynx in a clinical setting from the oral side with a single eye through a flexible endoscope. Views from the oral side through a flexible endoscope do not allow precise evaluation of the vertical level difference between the vocal folds, thickness of the affected fold, and separation of the vocal folds at the bottom during phonation

1.6.1   Glottal Insufficiency

Stroboscopic observation of the vocal folds reveals the presence of a glottal gap during phonation in the horizontal plane. Isshiki et al. reported that, in nearly half of UVFP patients, the affected fold is located superiorly to the normal fold during phonation [78]. In such a case, even when the glottis is apparently closed by stroboscopic observation, a glottal gap in the superior–inferior axis may exist. Thus, the glottal gap along the vertical plane must be evaluated using other methods.

1.6.2   Decrease in the Thickness of the Affected Vocal Fold

Asymmetry of vocal fold thickness cannot be assessed precisely by conventional stroboscopic observation from the oral side, just as in the evaluation of glottal insufficiency along the vertical plane. Thus, 3D evaluation of the laryngeal lumen is required for the diagnosis of UVFP.

1.6.3 Lowered Tension and Stiffness of the Vocal Fold

Cricothyroid muscle contraction results in elongation and elevates the anterior–posterior tension of the vocal fold. Thus, the CT muscle plays a major role in controlling the pitch of a generated sound. On the other hand, the TA muscle plays a key role in adjusting the stiffness of the cover and body of the vocal fold together with the CT muscle. The mucosal wave is elicited less without TA muscle contraction on the affected side or becomes aperiodical so that stroboscopic illumination fails to show the occurrence of the mucosal wave. The bowed appearance of the affected vocal fold during inhalation does not always indicate the presence of atrophy or flaccidity during phonation. Careful observation under stroboscopic illumination is indispensable.

1.6.4 Synkinetic Movement of the Affected Vocal Fold

Synkinesis, in general, is an unintentional movement accompanying a volitional movement and occurs after misdirected regeneration of nerve fibers. Laryngeal synkinesis is the result of misdirected and inappropriate reinnervation of the abductor muscle by adductor nerve fibers and vice versa [33]. One unfavorable synkinesis is abduction and thinning of the affected fold during phonation or adduction and thickening of the affected fold during inhalation. When the paralyzed vocal fold is flaccid, it may be blown up by the airstream to move passively upward and laterally. It is not possible to differentiate these by stroboscopic observation. EMG of the TA and PCA muscles is needed to confirm the presence of misdirected reinnervation. However, the performance of laryngeal EMG accompanies discomfort in patients; thus, only those scheduled for surgical treatment are indicated for EMG at the author's institution.

1.6.5 Over-adduction of the Normal Fold During Phonation

Adduction of the vocal fold on the unaffected side over the midline (over-adduction) during phonation has been mythologically thought to improve vocal function by decreasing the size of the glottal gap [79, 80]. However, according to the author's investigation [81, 82], over-adduction of the unaffected vocal fold had relatively little impact on vocal function.

References

1. Vogel PH. The innervations of the larynx of man and the dog. Am J Anat. 1952;90:427–47.
2. Sanudo JR, Maranillo E, Leon X, Mirapeix RM, Orus C, Quer M. An anatomical study of anastomoses between the laryngeal nerves. Laryngoscope. 1999;109:983–7.
3. Boles R, Fritzell B. Injury and repair of the recurrent laryngeal nerves in dogs. Laryngoscope. 1969;79:1405–18.

4. Shindo ML, Herzon GD, Hanson DG, Cain DJ, Sahgal V. Effects of denervation on laryngeal muscles: a canine model. Laryngoscope. 1992;102:663–9.
5. Woodson GE. Spontaneous laryngeal reinnervation after recurrent laryngeal or vagus nerve injury. Ann Otol Rhinol Laryngol. 2007;116:57–65.
6. Woodson G. Configuration of the glottis in laryngeal paralysis. II: animal experiments. Laryngoscope. 1993;103:1235–41.
7. Aronson AE, DeSanto LW. Adductor spastic dysphonia: three years after recurrent laryngeal nerve resection. Laryngoscope. 1983;93:1–8.
8. Schratzki H, Fritzell B. Treatment of spasmodic dysphonia by means of resection of the recurrent laryngeal nerve. Acta Otolaryngol. 1988;449:115–7.
9. Netterville JL, Stone RE, Rainey C, Zealear DL, Ossoff RH. Recurrent laryngeal nerve avulsion for treatment of spatic dysphonia. Ann Otol Rhinol Laryngol. 1991;100:10–4.
10. Crumley RL. Unilateral recurrent laryngeal nerve paralysis. J Voice. 1994;1:70–83.
11. Koufman JA, Walker FO, Joharji GM. The cricothyroid muscle does not influence vocal fold position in laryngeal paralysis. Laryngoscope. 1995;105:368–72.
12. Nomoto M, Yoshihara T, Kanda T, Kaneko T. Synapse formation by autonomic nerves in the previously denervated neuromuscular junctions of the feline intrinsic laryngeal muscles. Brain Res. 1991;539:276–86.
13. Nomoto M, Yoshihara T, Kanda T, Konno A, Kaneko T. Misdirected reinnervation in the feline intrinsic laryngeal muscles after long-term denervation. Acta Otolaryngol Suppl. 1993;506:71–4.
14. Sanders I, Wu B, Mu L, Li Y, Biller HF. The innervations of the human larynx. Arch Otolaryngol Head Neck Surg. 1993;119:934–9.
15. Wu BL, Sanders I, Mu L, Biller HF. The human communicating nerve. An extension of the external superior laryngeal nerve that innervates the vocal cord. Arch Otolaryngol Head Neck Surg. 1994;120:1321–8.
16. Crumley RC. Laryngeal synkinesis revisited. Ann Otol Rhinol Laryngol. 2000;109:365–71.
17. Gacek RR. Morphologic correlates for laryngeal reinnervation. Laryngoscope. 2001;111:1871–7.
18. Maranillo E, Vazquez T, Quer M, Niedenfuhr MR, Leon X, Viejo F, Parkin I, Sanudo JR. Potential structures that could be confused with a nonrecurrent inferior laryngeal nerve: an anatomical study. Laryngoscope. 2008;118:56–60.
19. Nasri S, Beizai P, Ye M, Sercarz JA, Kim YM, Berke GS. Cross-innervation of the thyroarytenoid muscle by a branch from the external division of the superior laryngeal nerve. Ann Otol Rhinol Laryngol. 1997;106:594–8.
20. Semon F. Clinical remarks. On the proclivity of the abductor fibers of the recurrent laryngeal nerve to become affected sooner than the adductor fibers or even exclusively; in cases of undoubted central or peripheral injury or disease of the roots or trunks of the pneumogastric, spinal accessory or recurrent nerves. Arch Laryngol. 1881;2:197–222.
21. Faaborg-Andersen K. The position of paretic vocal cords. Acta Otolaryngol. 1964;57:50–4.
22. Grossman M. Contribution to the mutural functional relationships of the muscles of the larynx. Arch Laryngol Rhinol. 1906;18:463–71.
23. Woodson GE. Configuration of the glottis in laryngeal paralysis. I: clinical study. Laryngoscope. 1993;103:1227–34.
24. Blitzer A, Jahn AF, Keider A. Semon's law revisited: an electromyographic analysis of laryngeal synkinesis. Ann Otol Rhinol Laryngol. 1996;105:764–9.
25. Maranillo E, Leon X, Orus C, Quer M, Sanudo JR. Variability in nerve patterns of the adductor muscle group supplied by the recurrent laryngeal nerve. Laryngoscope. 2005;115:358–62.
26. Brown MC, Holland RL, Hopkins WG. Motor nerve sprouting. Ann Rev Neurosci. 1981;4:17–42.
27. Damrose EJ, Huang RY, Blumin JH, Blackwell KE, Sercarz JA, Berke GS. Lack of evoked laryngeal electromyography response in patients with a clinical diagnosis of vocal cord paralysis. Ann Otol Rhinol Laryngol. 2001;110:815–9.

28. Siribodhi C, Sunderland W, Atkins JP, Bonner FJ. Electromyographic studies of laryngeal paralysis and regeneration of laryngeal motor nerves in dogs. Laryngoscope. 1963;73:148–63.
29. Hiroto I, Hirano M, Tomita H. Electromyographic investigations of human vocal cord paralysis. Ann Otol Rhinol Laryngol. 1968;77:296–304.
30. Tashiro T. Experimental studies of the reinnervation of larynx after accurate neurorrhaphy. Laryngoscope. 1972;82:225–36.
31. Ohyama M, Ueda N, Harvey JE, Mogi G, Ogura JH. Electrophysiologic study of reinnervated laryngeal motor units. Laryngoscope. 1972;82:237–51.
32. Satoh I, Harvey JH, Ogura JH. Impairment of function of the intrinsic laryngeal muscles after regeneration of the recurrent laryngeal nerve. Laryngoscope. 1974;84:53–66.
33. Crumley RL. Laryngeal synkinesis: its significance to the laryngologists. Ann Otol Rhinol Laryngol. 1989;98:87–92.
34. Flint PW, Downs DH, Coltrera MD. Laryngeal synkinesis following reinnervation in the rat: neuroanatomic and physiologic study using retrograde fluorescent tracers and electromyography. Ann Otol Rhinol Laryngol. 1991;100:797–806.
35. Nahm I, Shin T, Watanabe H, Maeyama T. Misdirected regeneration of injured recurrent laryngeal nerve in the cat. Am J Otolaryngol. 1993;14:43–8.
36. Min YB, Finnegan EM, Hoffman HT, Luschei ES, McCulloch TM. A preliminary study of the prognostic role of electromyography in laryngeal paralysis. Otolaryngol Head Neck Surg. 1994;111:770–5.
37. Wani MK, Woodson GE. Paroxysmal laryngospasm after laryngeal nerve injury. Laryngoscope. 1999;109:694–7.
38. Diamond J, Cooper E, Turner C, Macintyre L. Trophic regulation of nerve sprouting. Science. 1976;193:371–7.
39. Sunderland S, Swaney WE. The intraneural topography of the recurrent laryngeal nerve in man. Anat Rec. 1952;114:411–26.
40. Gacek RR, Malmgren LT, Lyon MJ. Localization of adductor and abductor motor nerve fibers to the larynx. Ann Otol Rhinol Laryngol. 1977;86:770–6.
41. Malmgren LT, Gacek RR. Acetylcholineesterase staining of fiber components in feline and human recurrent laryngeal nerve: topography of laryngeal motor fiber regions. Acta Otolaryngol. 1981;91:337–52.
42. Hisa Y, Koike S, Tadaki N, Bamba H, Shogaki K, Uno T. Neurotransmitters and neuromodulators involved in laryngeal innervation. Ann Otol Rhinol Laryngol. 1999;108:3–14.
43. Gordon JH, McCabe BF. The effect of accurate neurorrhaphy on reinnervation and return of laryngeal function. Laryngoscope. 1968;78:236–50.
44. Morledge DR, Lauvstad WA, Calcaterra TC. Delayed reinnervation of the paralyzed larynx. An experimental study in the dog. Arch Otolaryngol. 1973;37:291–3.
45. Eibling DE, Gross RD. Subglottic air pressure: a key component of swallowing efficiency. Ann Otol Rhinol Laryngol. 1996;105:253–8.
46. Carrau RL, Pou A, Eibling DE, Murry T. Laryngeal framework surgery for the management of aspiration. Head Neck. 1999;21:139–45.
47. Tabaee A, Murry T, Zschommler A, Desloge RB. Flexible endoscopic evaluation of swallowing with sensory testing in patients with unilateral vocal fold immobility: incidence and pathophysiology of aspiration. Laryngoscope. 2005;115:565–9.
48. Heitmiller RF, Tseng E, Jones B. Prevalence of aspiration and laryngeal penetration in patients with unilateral vocal fold motion impairment. Dysphagia. 2000;15:184–7.
49. Bhattacharyya N, Kotz T, Shapiro J. Dysphagia and aspiration with unilateral vocal cord immobility: incidence, characterization and response to surgical treatment. Ann Otol Rhinol Laryngol. 2002;111:672–9.
50. Smith E, Taylor M, Mendoza M, Barkmeier J, Lemke J, Hoffman H. Spasmodic dysphonia and vocal fold paralysis: outcomes of voice problems on work-related functioning. J Voice. 1998;12:223–32.

51. Benninger MS, Ahuja AS, Gardner G, Grywalski C. Assessing outcomes for dysphonic patients. J Voice. 1998;12:540–50.
52. Baba M, Natsugoe S, Shimada M, Nakano S, Noguchi Y, Kawachi K, Kusano C, Aikou T. Does hoarseness of voice from recurrent nerve paralysis after esophagectomy for carcinoma influence patient quality of life? J Am Coll Surg. 1999;188:231–6.
53. Fang TJ, Li HY, Glicklich RE, Chen YH, Wang PC, Chuang HF. Quality of life measures and predictors for adults with unilateral vocal cord paralysis. Laryngoscope. 2008;118:1837–41.
54. Isshiki N. Vocal efficiency index. In: Stevens KN, Hirano M, editors. Vocal fold physiology. Tokyo: University of Tokyo Press; 1981. p. 193–207.
55. Hirano M. Clinical examination of voice. Wien: Springer; 1981.
56. Lucero JC. Optimal glottal configuration for ease of phonation. J Voice. 1998;12:151–8.
57. Kobayashi J, Yumoto E, Hyodo M, Gyo K. Two-dimensional analysis of vocal fold vibration in unilaterally atrophied larynges. Laryngoscope. 2000;110:440–6.
58. Hirano M. Morphological structure of the vocal cord as a vibrator and its variations. Folia Phoniatr. 1974;26:89–94.
59. Yumoto E, Kadota Y, Kurokawa H. Thyroarytenoid muscle activity and infraglottic aspect of canine vocal fold vibration. Arch Otolaryngol Head Neck Surg. 1995;121:759–64.
60. Yanagi E, Slavit DH, McCaffrey TV. Study of phonation in the excised canine larynx. Otolaryngol Head Neck Surg. 1991;105:586–95.
61. Choi HS, Berke GS, Ye M, Kreiman J. Function of the thyroarytenoid muscle in a canine laryngeal model. Ann Otol Rhinol Laryngol. 1993;102:769–76.
62. Sloan SH, Berke GS, Gerratt BR, Kreiman J, Ye M. Determination of vocal fold mucosal wave velocity in an in vivo canine model. Laryngoscope. 1993;103:947–53.
63. Yumoto E, Kadota Y. Quantitative evaluation of the effects of thyroarytenoid muscle activity upon pliability of vocal fold mucosa in an in vivo canine model. Laryngoscope. 1997;107:266–72.
64. Sercarz JA, Berke GS, Ming YM, Gerratt BR, Natividad MN. Videostroboscopy of human vocal fold paralysis. Ann Otol Rhinol Laryngol. 1992;101:567–77.
65. Tanabe M, Isshiki N, Kitajima K. Vibratory pattern of the vocal cord in unilateral paralysis of the cricothyroid muscle. An experimental study. Acta Otolaryngol. 1972;74:339–45.
66. Isshiki N, Tanabe M, Ishizaka K, Broad D. Clinical significance of asymmetrical vocal cord tension. Ann Otol Rhinol Laryngol. 1977;86:58–66.
67. Maunsell R, Ouaknine M, Giovanni A, Crespo A. Vibratory pattern of vocal folds under tension asymmetry. Otolaryngol Head Neck Surg. 2006;135:438–44.
68. Yumoto E, Kurokawa H, Okamura H. Vocal fold vibration of the canine larynx: observation from an infraglottic view. J Voice. 1991;5:299–303.
69. Yumoto E, Kadota Y, Kurokawa H. Tracheal view of vocal fold vibration in excised canine larynx. Arch Otolaryngol Head Neck Surg. 1993;119:73–8.
70. Yumoto E, Kadota Y, Kurokawa H. Infraglottic aspect of canine vocal fold vibration: effect of increase of mean airflow rate and lengthening of vocal fold. J Voice. 1993;7:311–8.
71. Yumoto E, Kadota Y, Kurokawa H, Sasaki Y. Effects of vocal fold tension and thyroarytenoid activity on the infraglottic aspect of vocal fold vibration and glottal source sound quality. In: Fujimura O, Hirano M, editors. Vocal fold physiology: voice quality control. San Diego: Singular Publishing Group; 1995. p. 127–45.
72. Yumoto E, Kadota Y. Pliability of the vocal fold mucosa in relation to the mucosal upheaval during phonation. Arch Otolaryngol Head Neck Surg. 1998;124:897–902.
73. Hirano M, Yoshida T, Tanaka S. Vibratory behavior of human vocal folds viewed from below. In: Gauffin J, Hammarberg B, editors. Vocal fold physiology. Acoustic, perceptual, and physiological aspects of voice mechanism. San Diego: Singular Publishing Group; 1991. p. 1–6.
74. Yumoto E, Kadota Y, Mori T. Vocal fold vibration viewed from the tracheal side in living human beings. Otolaryngol Head Neck Surg. 1996;115:329–34.

75. Sanders I, Rai S, Han Y, Biller HF. Human vocalis contains distinct superior and inferior subcompartments: possible candidates for the two masses of vocal fold vibration. Ann Otol Rhinol Laryngol. 1998;107:826–33.
76. Sanders I, Han Y, Wang J, Biller H. Muscle spindles are concentrated in the superior vocalis subcompartment of the human thyroarytenoid muscle. J Voice. 1998;12:7–16.
77. Gray SD, Bielamowicz SA, Titze IR, Dove H, Ludlow C. Experimental approaches to vocal fold alteration: introduction to the minithyrotomy. Ann Otol Rhinol Laryngol. 1999;108:1–9.
78. Isshiki N, Ishikawa T. Diagnostic value of tomography in unilateral vocal cord paralysis. Laryngoscope. 1976;86:1573–8.
79. Yamada M, Hirano M. Recurrent laryngeal nerve paralysis. A 10-year review of 564 patients. Auris Nasus Larynx. 1983;10(Suppl):1–15.
80. Hirano M. Phonosurgery. Basic and clinical investigations. Otologia (Fukuoka). 1975;21:239–442.
81. Yumoto E, Nakano K, Oyamada Y. Relationship between 3D behavior of the unilaterally paralyzed larynx and aerodynamic vocal function. Acta Otolaryngol. 2003;123:274–8.
82. Yumoto E, Sanuki T, Minoda R, Kumai Y, Nishimoto K, Kodama N. Over-adduction of the unaffected vocal fold during phonation in the unilaterally paralyzed larynx. Acta Otolaryngol. 2014;134:744–52.

Chapter 2
Etiologies of Vocal Fold Paralysis and Conventional Surgical Procedures Used to Treat Paralytic Dysphonia

Abstract Modern imaging techniques including computed tomography, magnetic resonance imaging, and ultrasonography have advanced greatly over the last three decades, allowing the causes of vocal fold paralysis (VFP) to be established and improving the surgical treatment of patients with previously inoperable life-threatening diseases. However, VFP sometimes persists or even appears as a complication following surgery, resulting in breathy dysphonia and/or swallowing difficulties that affect postoperative quality of life (QOL) [1–4]. Thus, phonosurgical treatment of patients with paralytic dysphonia is important to improve QOL after treatment of the primary disease. In this chapter, the author reviews his experience in terms of the etiologies of VFP, the optimal surgical treatments for breathy dysphonia, and the vocal outcomes after surgery.

Keywords Etiologies of vocal fold paralysis • Vocal fold paralysis associated with surgery • Intracordal injection • Thyroplasty type I • Arytenoid adduction • Vocal function

2.1 Etiologies of Vocal Fold Paralysis

2.1.1 Diagnostic Procedures

The author examined 1,362 patients with VFP over 37 years, between October 1976 and December 2013. In this report, the 37 years are divided into three periods of 10 years and one period (the last) of 5 years; the periods are: October 1976 to December 1986, January 1987 to December 1997, October 1998 to December 2008, and January 2009 to December 2013. Data on patients with VFP, who were examined by the author at Ehime University Hospital (Ehime, Japan), were collected between October 1976 and December 1997; data on patients seen at Kumamoto University Hospital (Kumamoto, Japan) were collected from October 1998 to December 2013. Since the author moved from Ehime University to Kumamoto University in October 1998, data from the interval between January and September 1988 were not included. Patients with vocal fold immobility attributable to invasive laryngeal or hypopharyngeal cancer, subluxation of the cricoarytenoid joint,

© Springer Japan 2015

E. Yumoto, *Pathophysiology and Surgical Treatment of Unilateral Vocal Fold Paralysis*, DOI 10.1007/978-4-431-55354-0_2

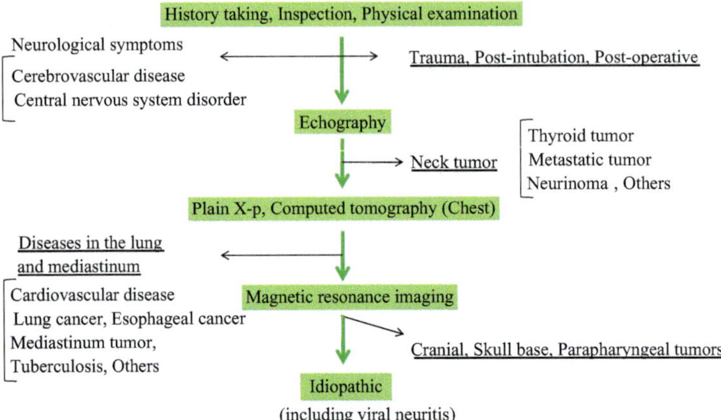

Fig. 2.1 A flow chart to aid correct diagnosis of the cause of vocal fold paralysis

adhesion of the posterior glottis, or rheumatoid arthritis-derived cricoarytenoid joint fixation were excluded.

Figure 2.1 presents a flow chart indicating how the cause of VFP should be investigated. History taking and physical examination, including endoscopy of the head-and-neck region, are essential in this context. Other modalities, including neck ultrasonography, chest radiography, chest computed tomography (CT), and magnetic resonance imaging of the cranial cavity and the skull base to the parapharyngeal space, should be requested when indicated. If such investigations fail to define the cause of VFP, the patient should be followed up for at least 3 months, at which time a thorough examination should be repeated. An idiopathic diagnosis should only be made when the underlying cause of VFP cannot be established at the end of the follow-up period.

Viral infections can cause VFP, but such infections are not easy to confirm. Antiviral antibody titers are not routinely measured, because patients do not visit hospitals immediately after symptom onset. The presence of vesicles in the laryngo-pharyngeal region on the same side as the VFP may suggest that viral infection is in play. Herpes zoster virus, herpes simplex virus, and other viruses have been reported to cause VFP [5–10]. Thus, VFP patients in idiopathic categories may include those with virus-related VFP.

2.1.2   *The Author's Experience*

Table 2.1 shows the numbers of male and female patients seen at the author's institutions, by decade of patient age. The patients included 775 males (56.9 %) and 587 females (43.1 %), ranging in age from 2 months to 93 years, with a mean age of 60.3 years (61.1 years in males and 59.1 years in females). The numbers of male patients increased from the fifth decade of patient age, peaking in the seventh decade, and the numbers of female patients increased from the fourth decade, peaking in the seventh decade. The numbers of female patients in the second, fourth, and fifth decades of life were greater than those of male patients in the corresponding decades. The female preponderance in these decades of age may be associated with the higher incidence of thyroid disease in females. Statistical analysis was performed using the chi-squared test. A difference was considered significant when the P value was less than 0.05. Unilateral VFP (UVFP) was evident in 1,221 patients (89.6 %), whereas 141 patients (10.4 %) presented with bilateral VFP. Of the 1,221 patients with UVFP, 835 patients (68.4 %) had left-side paralysis and 386 patients (31.6 %) had right-side paralysis; the incidence of UVFP on the left side was twice that on the right. Twenty-three patients were lost to follow-up, and their data were excluded from analysis.

Table 2.2 shows the numbers of patients who developed VFP not associated with and associated with surgery in the four study periods. The numbers of patients who developed VFP after surgery were significantly higher in Groups 2–4 than in Group 1 ($P < 0.0001$).

Table 2.1 Numbers of male and female patients with unilateral vocal fold paralysis by decade of patient age

Age	Male	Female	Total
0–9	12	7	19
10–19	8	10	18
20–29	27	17	44
30–39	32	44	76
40–49	66	69	135
50–59	143	124	267
60–69	248	151	399
70–79	188	122	310
80–89	50	40	90
90~	2	2	4
Total	775(56.9 %)	587(43.1 %)	1,362

Table 2.2 Number of patients with vocal fold paralysis unrelated to and related to surgery in the four successive periods

	Group 1 Oct. 1976 – Dec.1986	Group 2 Jan. 1987 – Dec. 1997	Group 3 Oct. 1998 – Dec. 2008	Group 4 Jan. 2009 – Dec. 2013	Total
Not related to surgery	162 (71.4 %)	115 (48.1 %)	289 (55.2 %)	181 (51.7 %)	747 (55.8 %)
Related to surgery	65 (28.6 %)	124 (51.9 %)	234 (44.7 %)	169 (48.3 %)	592 (44.2 %)
Total	227	239	523	350	1,339

P < 0.0001
P < 0.0001
P < 0 .0001

In Tables 2.3 and 2.4, patients are classified by cause of VFP; the former table shows the VFP etiologies of 747 patients with diseases unrelated to surgery, and the latter table shows the etiologies of surgery-associated disease in 592 patients. Among patients with surgery-unrelated paralysis, 227 (30.4 %) had upper thorax disorders, including malignant neoplasms of the lung and esophagus. The numbers of patients who developed VFP after diagnosis of tuberculosis fell from eight in Group 1 to zero or one in the other groups. Thyroid cancer was the most frequent cause of VFP among patients with neck lesions, and the incidence of such disease was significantly higher in Group 1 than in Group 3 (P=0.0400). Idiopathic VFP was evident in 265 of the total of 1,339 patients (19.8 %) and in 35.4 % of the 747 patients in whom VFP was not associated with a surgical procedure.

Most neck surgical causes of VFP were associated with surgery used to treat benign and malignant thyroid tumors. The numbers of VFP patients after thyroid surgery were 24 (36.9 %) of 65 in Group 1, 52 (41.9 %) of 124 in Group 2, 87

Table 2.3 Etiologies of 604 patients with vocal fold paralysis not related to surgery

		Group 1 Oct. 1976 – Dec.1986	Group 2 Jan. 1987 – Dec. 1997	Group 3 Oct. 1998 – Dec. 2008	Group 4 Jan. 2009 – Dec. 2013	Total
Head	Brain tumor	1	0	7	2	10
	Cerebrovascular disease	1	7	22	3	33
	Nasopharyngeal cancer	2	0	2	1	5
	Others	4	0	10	7	21
	Subtotal	8	7	41	13	69
Neck	Thyroid cancer	16	13 *	51	31	111
	Metastatic tumor	9	4	5	9	27
	Trauma	7	5	2	1	15
	Others	4	0	11	8	23
	Subtotal	36	22	69	49	176
Thorax	Esophageal cancer	10	9	19	8	46
	Lung cancer	20	20	30	19	89
	Tuberculosis	8	1	0	1	10
	Other lung disease	4	0	1	0	5
	Metastatic tumor	3	0	9	7	19
	Mediastinal tumor	5	8	6	6	25
	Heart disease	3	0	0	0	3
	Aortic arch aneurysm	0	1	10	5	16
	Others	2	3	5	4	14
	Subtotal	55	42	80	50	227
	Polyneuritis	4	2	4	0	10
	Idiopathic	59	42	95	69	265
	Total	162	115	289	181	747

*: P=0.0400

Table 2.4 Etiologies of 459 patients with vocal fold paralysis related to surgery

		Group 1 Oct. 1976 – Dec.1986	Group 2 Jan. 1987 – Dec. 1997	Group 3 Oct. 1998 – Dec. 2008	Group 4 Jan. 2009 – Dec. 2013	Total
Head	Brain tumor	1	1	4	3	9
	Skull base tumor	0	3	4	0	7
	Cerebral aneurysm	0	0	7	2	9
	Others	0	0	2	2	4
	Subtotal	1	4	17	7	29
Neck	Benign thyroid tumor	11	23	9	6	49
	Thyroid cancer	13	29	78	44	164
	Neurinoma	0	2	4	2	8
	Others	6	8	14	4	32
	Subtotal	30	62	105	56	253
Thorax	Esophageal cancer	5	10	39	27	81
	Lung cancer	7	5	6	22	40
	Tuberculosis	2	0	0	0	2
	Mediastinal tumor	1	2	1	2	6
	Heart disease	1	8	7	4	20
	Aortic arch aneurysm	0	6	21	22	49
	Others	4	6	3	6	19
	Subtotal	20	37	77	83	217
Post-intubation		14	21	35	23	93
Total		65	124	234	169	592

*: P<0.0001 for comparisons between Groups 2 and 3 and between Groups 2 and 4
**: P=0.0003 and 0.0006 for comparisons between Groups 1 and 3 and between Groups 1 and 4, respectively
***: P=0.0363
****: P=0.0123 and 0.00854 for comparisons between Groups 2 and 4 and between Groups 3 and 4, respectively
*****: P=0.0252 for comparison between Groups 2 and 4

(37.2 %) of 234 in Group 3, and 50 (30.0 %) of 169 in Group 4. Thus, the incidence of VFP after thyroid surgery was consistent over the past four periods. The incidence of developing VFP after surgery to treat benign thyroid diseases was significantly lower in Groups 3 and 4 than in Groups 1 and 2 (please note the P values in Table 2.4). The incidence of VFP developing after surgery to treat lung cancer was higher in Group 4 compared to Groups 2 and 3 (the P values were 0.0123 and 0.00854, respectively). The incidence of postesophagectomy VFP was likewise higher in Groups 3 and 4 than in Groups 1 and 2 (the P value for the comparison between Groups 2 and 3 was 0.0363, thus statistically significant). Although statistical significance was not attained, the P values for comparisons between Groups 1 and 3 and Groups 2 and 4 were 0.0952 and 0.0597, respectively. Surgical intervention to treat aortic arch aneurysms was associated with an increased VFP incidence when Groups 2 and 4 were compared (P=0.0252). In general, surgical treatments for patients suffering from previously inoperable life-threatening diseases have progressed over the years, and it is thus more important than ever to improve postoperative QOL via phonosurgical treatment of severe breathy dysphonia.

2.2 Phonosurgical Procedures to Improve Paralytic Dysphonia

2.2.1 Historical Review

Figure 2.2 presents details of phonosurgical treatments for paralytic dysphonia, depending on the purpose of such treatment. Intracordal injections, insertion of fascia, and thyroplasty type I (Type I method) seek to increase the mass of the vocal fold. The type I method also effectively medializes the vocal fold, depending on the size and shape of the inserted material. Arytenoid adduction and various modifications thereof have been reported to move the affected vocal fold to the median position and to correct any vertical mismatch between vocal folds. Furthermore, reconstruction of laryngeal muscle innervation includes direct anastomosis of the severed ends of the recurrent laryngeal nerve (RLN), interpositioning of a free nerve graft between such severed ends, anastomosis between the proximal end of the ansa

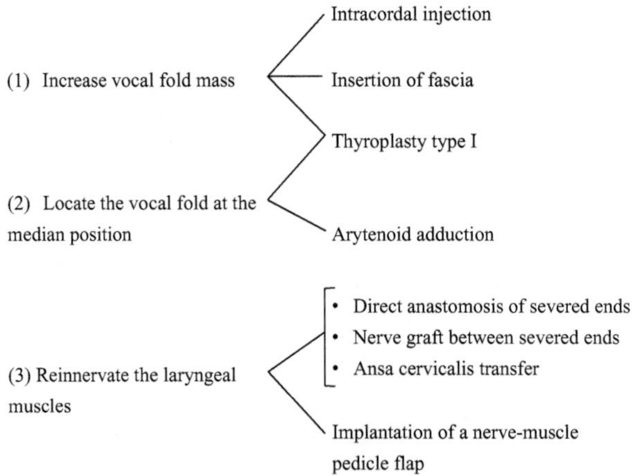

Fig. 2.2 Classification of phonosurgical treatments depending on the purpose of each method

cervicalis nerve (ACN) and the distal end of the RLN (AC transfer), and implantation of a nerve–muscle pedicle flap (NMP) utilizing the ACN. The purposes of these reinnervation methods are recovery of vocal fold mass and tension and median localization of the affected vocal fold.

2.2.2 *Intracordal Injection and Fascia Insertion*

In 1911, Brunings first described intracordal injection of paraffin to treat paralytic dysphonia [11]. Unfortunately, adverse effects including tissue migration and granulation developed, and paraffin is no longer used. Many other intracordal materials have been described, but no widely accepted injection material has yet been defined. An ideal injection material should be biologically inert (i.e., incapable of stimulating a foreign body or allergic reaction), be stable in the injected location (i.e., not exhibiting tissue migration), be resistant to resorption (i.e., absorption is minimal after injection), and not inhibit development of a mucosal wave. Both Teflon [12–14] and silicon [15, 16] were used as injection materials after paraffin was abandoned. However, Teflon caused frequent granuloma formation because of foreign body reaction and tended to migrate from the injection site, being excreted into the airway [17–19]. Silicon also exhibited disadvantages, including a foreign body reaction (although less severe than that associated with Teflon) and migration from and diffusion within the tissue [20, 21]. Thus, these two materials are no longer popular.

In the time since Ford and Bless introduced atelocollagen (bovine collagen from which antigenic telopeptides have been removed) as an injection material in 1986 [22], many other materials have been considered. These include autologous fat [23, 24], minced autologous fascia [25, 26], extracellular components of human skin [27, 28], calcium hydroxyl apatite [29–31], and hyaluronic acid [32, 33]. In Japan, autologous fat injection has become popular [34, 35]. Autologous fat cannot cause an allergic reaction, and is not associated with any danger of transmittal of unknown infectious agents. However, injected fat tends to be absorbed quite quickly, and it is difficult to predict how much will be absorbed. To reduce resorption, Tamura et al. [36] included basic fibroblast growth factor with the fat injection. Other methods used to reduce resorption include purification of harvested fat [37–39] and the use of a buccal fat pad rather than subcutaneous abdominal fat [40]. To the best of the author's knowledge, no ideal injectable material is yet available.

Tsunoda et al. [41–43] devised a method in which a sheet of fascia was inserted between the body and the cover of the vocal fold. Nishiyama et al. [44, 45] developed this method further by creating a roll of fascia to augment the effect thereof. Although the cited authors aimed to medialize the affected vocal fold, the long-term results (12 months after surgery) were not satisfactory, as exemplified by averages of only an 11 s maximum phonation time (MPT) and a 500 mL/s mean airflow rate (MFR) in eight patients with paralytic dysphonia. The injection laryngoplasties and fascia transplantation described above were performed through the laryngeal lumen, and thus, no skin incision was required [46].

2.2.3 *Type I Thyroplasty (Medialization Thyroplasty)*

The purpose of the type I method is to facilitate glottal closure during phonation by increasing the mass of the affected vocal fold. Payr first developed this idea in 1915 [47], and many modifications have since been proposed [48–51]. These methods are effective in reducing glottal insufficiency, but it is not possible to adjust the medial pressure finely during operation. In 1974, Isshiki et al. [52] proposed the type I method for augmenting the affected vocal fold and shifting it medially by pressing the fold through a window in the thyroid ala set at the level of the fold. Custom-designed silicon blocks were used as insertion materials. Surgery was performed under local anesthesia so that the patient's voice could be monitored during the operation. The method was used to treat paralytic dysphonia, and it was possible to adjust the pressure intraoperatively by varying the thickness of the silicon block [53].

It is necessary to construct a window at the level of the vocal fold during phonation. Isshiki et al. [52, 53] developed a method for predicting the vertical level of the vocal fold. Misplacement of the window, often cranially to the vocal fold, is one of the most frequent causes of treatment failure. Methods used to confirm correct window positioning are (in addition to precise choice of window location using the Isshiki approach): [52, 53] piercing of the laryngeal lumen with a 30 G needle [54] and pressing the tissue through the window using a lacrimal duct bougie [55] under endoscopic guidance from inside the airway. Isshiki et al. [56–58] adjusted silicon thickness intraoperatively, thereby prolonging the operative time. To address this problem, prefabricated materials are currently available in several sizes. In 1998, McCulloch et al. [59] reported that polytetrafluoroethylene (Gore-Tex®; PTFE) sheet could serve as an insertion material. PTFE sheet affords several advantages compared to other insertion materials as it is easily adjustable and biologically inert and only a relatively small window is required. However, the adductory force produced upon insertion of a large portion of stiff material cannot be attained by employing folded Gore-Tex® sheet; the material is too pliable. Figure 2.3 shows the author's modification of the type I method using a PTFE sheet.

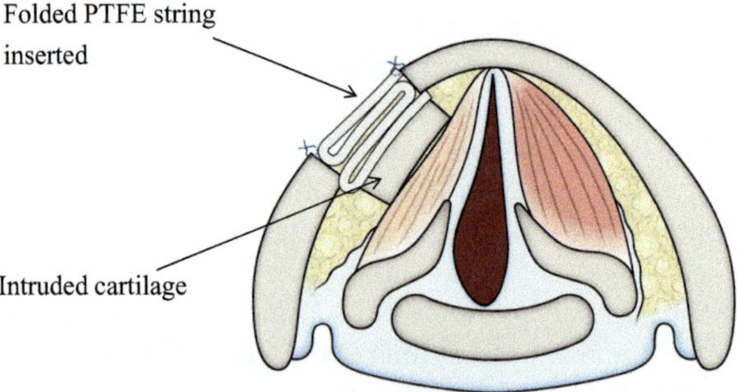

Fig. 2.3 Type I thyroplasty using polytetrafluoroethylene (Gore-Tex®, PTFE) sheet as an insertion material

2.2.4   Arytenoid Adduction

Although the type I method and intracordal injection can reduce the glottal gap, any effect is usually limited to the anterior part of the glottis. Arytenoid adduction (AA) is performed to close the glottal gap between the vocal processes (the posterior glottal gap) during phonation. In 1948, Morrison developed a method by which the affected vocal fold could be moved toward the midline; the arytenoid cartilage was glided medially along the upper border of the cricoid cartilage after separating the two cartilages [60]. The procedure was considered invasive, and it was technically difficult to locate and fix the arytenoid cartilage at the right position. In 1966, Montgomery developed the cricoarytenoid arthrodesis technique, in which the arytenoid was fixed onto the cricoid cartilage using a custom-made pin via a laryngofissure approach [61]. The vocal fold mucosa inevitably became cicatricial after mucosal incision (a consequence of the laryngofissure approach), and the procedure was rather invasive. In 1978, Isshiki et al. [62] developed a method by which the affected vocal fold is rotated at the median position by pulling on the muscular process of the arytenoid cartilage (Fig. 2.4). This method affords several advantages compared to earlier approaches; the laryngeal lumen is not opened (i.e., the vocal fold mucosa is not injured), the operation can be performed under local anesthesia, the patient's voice can be monitored during surgery, and the arytenoid cartilage is readily fixed at the median position. AA has therefore become popular and is now the treatment of choice for paralytic dysphonia. Several key features of AA are described in the following paragraphs.

2.2.4.1   Location of the Muscular Process of the Arytenoid

In the Isshiki method, the connection between the superior cornu of the thyroid cartilage and thyrohyoid ligament is released, and then the cricothyroid (CT) joint is separated. The thyroid ala is pulled and rotated to open the paraglottic

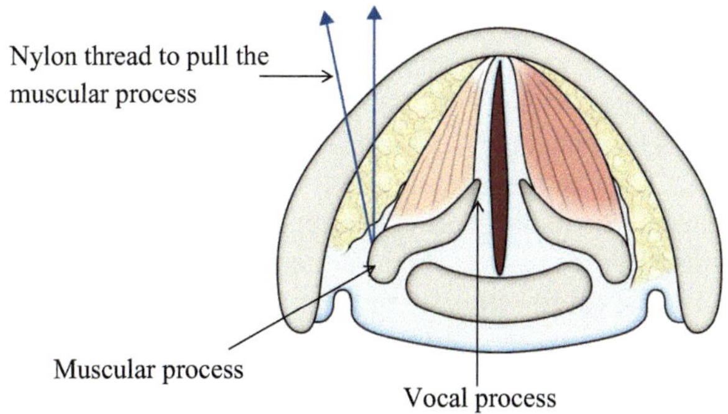

Fig. 2.4 Arytenoid adduction to locate the affected vocal fold at the midline

space. The muscular process is located about 1 cm cranially from the CT joint. It is important to not injure the pyriform sinus (PS) mucosa, which partly overhang this muscular process. It is easy to identify the muscular process if the inner surface of the thyroid cartilage is subperichondrially elevated and the paraglottic space is opened widely.

Several modifications of the method have been reported in efforts to approach the muscular process without separating the CT joint. Iwamura et al. [63], Sonoda et al. [64], and Tokashiki et al. [65] made a window in the thyroid ala more posteriorly as it was larger than that used in the type I method, to locate and pull the lateral cricoarytenoid (LCA) muscle or the muscular process anteriorly. Maragos made a posterior window in the thyroid ala and located the muscular process after elevation of the inner perichondrium together with the PS mucosa [66]. Su et al. [67] separated the thyroid cartilage 5 mm away from the midline, elevated the inner perichondrium posteriorly, and traced the LCA muscle to attain the muscular process. Care should be taken to not injure the PS mucosa when employing these modified techniques. The author basically used the Isshiki method to identify the muscular process but avoided opening the cricoarytenoid (CA) joint. Thus, pulling of the muscular process did not result in an anterior shift of the arytenoid cartilage.

2.2.4.2 Separation of the Cricothyroid Joint

The modified methods described above do not involve CT joint separation. If the CT joint is in fact separated, anterior pulling on the muscular process rotates the vocal fold medially and may impart a certain amount of force that pulls on the thyroid cartilage where the anterior end of the vocal fold attaches posteriorly, resulting in a somewhat shorter vocal fold. However, based on the author's experience, such posterior traction of the thyroid cartilage is not significant in production of vocal fold vibration.

2.2.4.3 Management of the Cricoarytenoid Joint

In the method by Isshiki et al. [53], the CA joint is opened to identify the joint-side surface of the arytenoid cartilage. This step ensures proper localization of the muscular process and is recommended to those who are not familiar with AA. However, opening of the CA joint is not necessary to locate the muscular process if the surgeon is experienced. The author locates the muscular process without opening the CA joint, because posterior support for the arytenoid is lost when the joint is opened and the affected vocal fold becomes shorter than that of the contralateral fold by virtue of anterior pulling on the muscular process. Such imbalance creates asymmetry in vocal fold tension, and the shortened fold becomes bowed. Such changes negatively influence postoperative voice [68].

2.2.4.4   Direction of Threads Used to Pull the Muscular Process

Isshiki et al. [53] pulled two threads tied to the muscular process anteriorly and fixed them onto the surface of the thyroid ala. However, theoretically, the threads should be pulled in the direction of the LCA muscle (i.e., toward the cricoid cartilage). In fact, Su et al. [69] reported that traction on the muscular process, applied toward the cricoid cartilage, yielded better voice results than did traction toward the lower part of the thyroid ala. Furthermore, in addition to the anterior pulling of the muscular process, Woodson et al. [70] tied a suture between the muscular process and the inferior cornu of the thyroid cartilage to prevent anterior tilting of the arytenoid, which may develop upon loss of posterior support by the posterior cricoarytenoid (PCA) muscle.

2.2.4.5   Laryngeal Edema After Surgery

Edematous changes in the laryngeal lumen, on the operated side, develop after surgery, but as long as the vocal fold on the unaffected side exhibits physiological movement, such mucosal swelling does not affect respiratory function. However, several authors have reported that 2–5 % of patients require tracheostomy after AA to relieve respiratory distress [71–74]. To prevent such a complication, the author pays special attention to certain issues during surgery. These are: precise and gentle management of each step of the procedure, complete hemostasis during manipulation of tissue (especially the severed edges of muscles), and intravenous administration of 500 mg hydrocortisone sodium succinate just before the paraglottic space is entered.

2.2.5   Combination of AA with the Type I Method or Intracordal Injection

The type I method or intracordal injection is usually indicated if the glottal gap during phonation is small, whereas AA is performed to close a larger gap, especially a posterior glottal gap. Because of the easy accessibility of the thyroid ala, the type I method is frequently used to treat paralytic dysphonia. Figure 2.5 shows laryngeal images obtained after AA (left) and the use of the type I method (right) on a single excised larynx. Arrows indicate the location of the tip of the vocal process. A silicon block (the insert in the left picture of Fig. 2.5) was used to push both the membranous and cartilaginous parts of the vocal fold medially. As indicated by the arrows, AA caused adduction of the vocal process, and the membranous part became concave (like a bow). On the other hand, the use of the type I method caused the vocal fold to bulge, but the vocal process was not sufficiently adducted, although the posterior part was pushed medially by a custom-designed silicon block [75].

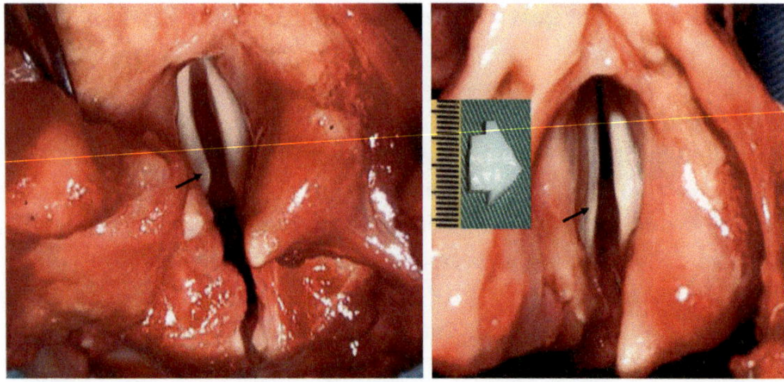

Fig. 2.5 Laryngeal images after performance of arytenoid adduction (*left*) and thyroplasty type I (*right*) on a single excised larynx. *Arrows* indicate the tip of the vocal process. The insert shows a silicon block designed to push together the anterior and posterior parts of the vocal fold (Citation: Ref. [75])

Therefore, a combination of AA and the type I method is often applied [65, 76–78]. Similarly, AA can also be combined with intracordal injection to enhance medialization of the membranous part [79].

Zeitels et al. [80, 81] developed adduction arytenopexy, which simulates the natural gliding and inward rocking that occurs upon normal adduction. The arytenoid body is positioned on the medial aspect of the cricoid facet. The cited authors combined the type I method with adduction arytenopexy. During adduction arytenopexy, the CT joint is separated, triggering anteromedial rotation of the thyroid ala. Zeitels et al. [82] sought to compensate for this unwanted effect by placing a suture between the inferior cornu and the anterior part of the cricoid, thus simulating cricothyroid muscle contraction to increase the tension on and the length of the vocal fold on the affected side (the process was termed cricothyroid subluxation). In 1990, cricothyroid approximation (thyroplasty type IV [52]) was used to increase the tension of the vocal fold, and positive effects on voice after AA were reported [83].

2.2.6   *Remobilization of an Affected Vocal Fold*

As described in Chap. 1, even when the intrinsic laryngeal muscles are reinnervated, physiological vocal fold movement does not recover. Isshiki switched a cartilage–muscle flap harvested from the CT muscle to the muscular process to achieve adduction of the vocal fold. In acute experiments with dogs, a degree of mobility (about one-third that of normal) was noted. The method was tested on one patient, but no adductive movement was observed postoperatively [84]. Nonomura et al. [85] sutured the CT muscle to the LCA muscle of the unilaterally paralyzed canine larynx in an effort to perform dynamic reconstruction. Firing of the superior laryngeal nerve served as a trigger, and contraction of the CT muscle served as the driving force. Recovery of adductive movement in an affected vocal fold was reported in 17 of 18 dogs immediately after suturing. In addition, electrophysiological and histological examinations revealed that the external branch of the superior laryngeal nerve (SLN) had reinnervated the LCA muscle [85]. The method was used to treat seven patients, and some adductive movement was evident in four [86]. However, such favorable results have not been confirmed.

2.2.7   Reinnervation of the Laryngeal Muscles

Figure 2.6 shows four different methods used for reinnervation of the paralyzed larynx. Direct suturing of the severed ends of the RLN is best, if possible. However, direct suturing is seldom feasible in clinical settings, except when the nerve defect is less than 5 mm in length. The second method involves interposition of a piece of foreign nerve between the ends of the RLN. A section of the great auricular nerve (GAN) is commonly used for this purpose, because the GAN and RLN lie close together and are similar in diameter, and minimal adverse effects are created at the donor site. The third method is nerve transfer, in which the ACN is sutured to the

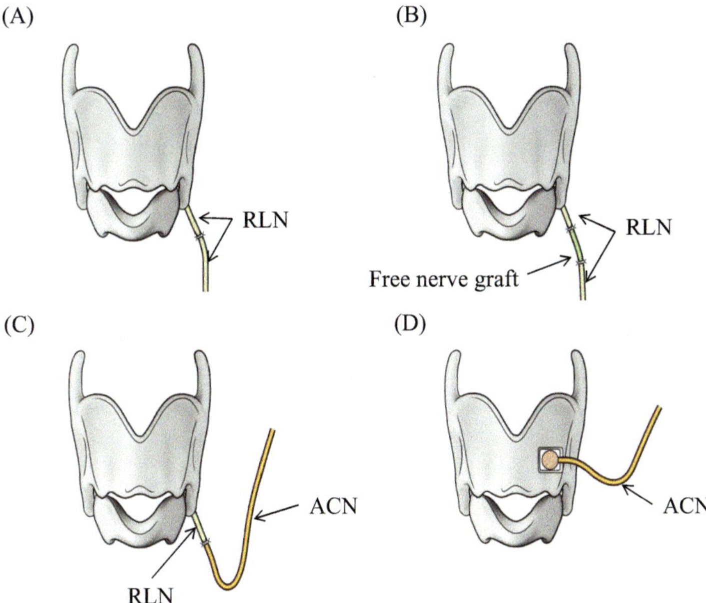

Fig. 2.6 Schematic representation of reconstruction methods used for laryngeal reinnervation. (**A**) Direct suturing of the severed ends of the recurrent laryngeal nerve (RLN). (**B**) Free nerve interposition between the severed ends of the RLN. (**C**) Ansa cervicalis nerve (ACN)-to-RLN anastomosis. (**D**) Nerve-muscle pedicle (NMP) flap implantation in the thyroarytenoid muscle. The NMP flap is harvested from the ACN and the sternohyoid muscle

peripheral end of the RLN (when the central end is unavailable for reconstruction). The fourth method is implantation of a nerve–muscle pedicle (NMP) flap (when the peripheral end of the RLN is unavailable), although this method has not yet been shown to be useful in clinical settings. The original innervation from the RLN is reconstructed via direct suture and nerve interposition, but aberrant regeneration of nerve fibers may occur. Interposition of a free nerve graft requires two sutures, whereas nerve transfer requires only a single suture (between the ACN and RLN). Reinnervation occurs in muscle in which an NMP flap is implanted. When the ACN on the affected side is unavailable, the ACN on the unaffected side can be utilized for nerve transfer and in the NMP flap implantation method.

2.2.7.1 Immediate Reconstruction of Laryngeal Muscle Innervation

Immediate reconstruction of the RLN via direct suturing, nerve interposition, or nerve transfer during extirpation of neck malignancies affords excellent vocal outcomes [87–90]. Yumoto et al. [89] followed up the vocal functions of 22 patients for 9 months after resection of primary lesions and tumors involving the RLN. Immediate reconstruction of the RLN was performed in nine patients (Group 1). Nine patients opted to not undergo phonosurgical procedures (Group 2), and the remaining four underwent AA immediately after tumor extirpation (Group 3). Group 1 patients showed significantly better vocal function than Group 2 patients with regard to all of the stroboscopic, aerodynamic, and acoustic results. Group 3 patients had gaps of varying degrees along the membranous vocal fold. Although the harmonics-to-noise ratio (HNR) [91], shimmer, and MPT of Group 3 were comparable to those of Group 1, other parameters (jitter, MFR, glottal gap) were poorer than in Group 1. Tanaka et al. [92] harvested a piece of the sternohyoid muscle 1×2 cm in size, with the ACN connected, and inserted the flap into the paraglottic space after extirpation of thyroid cancer with concomitant removal of the RLN. The voice of seven of nine such patients improved; the MPT was longer than 10 s and the MFR less than 200 mL/s. The cited authors sought to reinnervate the thyroarytenoid (TA) and LCA muscles and to ensure that the vocal fold would be pressed medially by a large muscle flap. Although vocal function improved over time, no electromyographic evidence of reinnervation was presented. Laryngeal edema occurred in one patient, and a temporary tracheostomy was necessary. Thus, insertion of a large mass into the paraglottic space may enhance edematous changes in the vocal fold and the arytenoid mucosa.

2.2.7.2 Reinnervation of Laryngeal Muscles After Onset of Vocal Fold Paralysis

In patients with paralytic dysphonia, Tucker [93, 94] implanted an NMP flap, harvested from the superior belly of the omohyoid muscle, into the TA muscle through a window in the thyroid ala and reported voice improvements after surgery. Later, the cited author combined the type I method and the NMP technique and reported better results than the type I method alone [95–97]. May and Beery also implanted an NMP flap into the LCA muscle, and vocal function improved in 22 of 29 (76 %) patients [98]. The voice improvements were ascribed to an increase in tone and/or slight changes in vocal fold configuration, allowing the normal side to oppose the affected side during phonation. In addition, it was suggested that apart from a reinnervation effect, the implanted muscle added bulk to the paralyzed vocal fold, and fibrosis of the inserted muscle may have assisted vocal fold positioning near the midline. In 2003, Maronian et al. [99] performed NMP flap implantation on three patients and reported electromyographic evidence of reinnervation of the TA muscle in one. However, objective assessment of vocal function was not performed. To the best of the author's knowledge, no studies except those reviewed above have used NMP flaps.

In 1986, Crumley et al. [100–102] reported good results after nerve transfer (ACN-to-RLN anastomosis). Gelfoam was injected after nerve transfer to ensure short-term results because such transfer usually begins to take effect only several months after the procedure. Lorenz et al. [103] performed this procedure on 46 patients and evaluated voice quality in 21 patients using the Consensus Auditory–Perceptual Evaluation of Voice (CAPE-V) scale, where 0 is normal and 100 severely abnormal. The severities of hoarseness and breathiness were 61.3 and 53.3 before surgery and improved to 37.9 and 43.8, respectively, by 18 months after surgery. Thus, despite improvements during long-term follow-up, postoperative voice quality did not regain normal status. Olson et al. [104] reported similar results after nerve transfer. Paniello [105] performed laryngeal reinnervation via anastomosis between the RLN and hypoglossal nerve of nine patients and reported excellent voice quality upon acoustic analysis in five patients followed up for 1 year. However, the method has two disadvantages: the use of the hypoglossal nerve disturbed the articulatory and swallowing function of the tongue (albeit slightly) and a segment of the peripheral RLN longer than 3 cm was required for tension-free nerve suturing. Su et al. [106] implanted the ACN, without a muscle fragment, into the TA muscle through a window of the thyroid ala in 10 patients. Eight patients exhibited voice improvement after surgery, and electromyographic evidence of recruitment during phonation was obtained for four patients. Thus, the data show that reinnervation of laryngeal muscle(s) is useful for improving vocal function in patients suffering from breathy dysphonia caused by unilateral VFP.

Paniello et al. [107] reported on a multicenter randomized trial comparing framework surgeries (the type I method alone or combined with AA) with nerve transfer (anastomosis of the ACN with the RLN). At 12 months after surgery, both groups exhibited significant improvements in vocal function compared to that before surgery, although most results were not within normal ranges. No significant difference in vocal function was evident between the two groups. Patient age affected vocal function in the nerve transfer group in that patients less than 52 years of age enjoyed significantly better results than older patients. Thus, it was suggested that laryngeal reinnervation should be used in younger patients, whereas framework surgeries should be favored for older patients. However, only very small numbers of patients (12 in each group) were studied; thus, the effectiveness of reinnervation in older patients should be examined with larger numbers of patients to establish definitive indications for use with regard to patient age.

2.2.7.3   Combination of Reinnervation and Framework Surgery

Tucker combined the type I method with the NMP technique and reported better results compared to the use of the former technique alone, as described in the previous section [97]. Chhetri et al. [108] combined ACN-to-RLN anastomosis with AA in ten patients and compared their vocal outcomes to those of nine patients who underwent AA alone. Both groups significantly improved after surgery. However, postoperative voice quality in the reinnervation group (a mean rating of 2.9 on a seven-point scale, where 1 indicated normal quality and 7 indicated severely abnormal quality) was still far from normal. One reason for such an unsatisfactory result may be that the follow-up periods ranged from 3 to 36 months. Chhetri et al. [108] found no significant difference between groups. Hassan et al. [109] assessed the long-term vocal functions of nine patients who underwent ACN-to-RLN anastomosis and AA. All parameters examined (MPT, pitch range, HNR, perceptual voice quality) improved significantly soon after surgery and continued to improve over a 24-month period. However, the work did not include a patient group undergoing AA alone; thus, it remains unclear whether a combination of reinnervation and AA affords better vocal function than AA alone or AA combined with the type I method or intracordal injection.

2.2.8   Vocal Function After Application of the Abovementioned Methods

Table 2.5 summarizes postoperative vocal function outcomes reported in the recent literature. Data on acoustic analysis are not included because the measurements obtained depend on the recording device and environment used, the vowel analyzed, and the analytical software algorithm employed. Vocal function clearly improved after injection of autologous fat or fascia and after the use of the type I method, but never became normal. Combinations of AA with the type I method or an injection method yielded better vocal function compared to that afforded by use of the latter techniques alone. Zeitels et al. [80–82] and Tokashiki et al. [65] reported that vocal function fell within the normal ranges of MPT and MFR. However, neither report evaluated perceptual voice quality.

2.3   The Author's Experience During the 15 Years Between 1986 and 2001

The author performed intracordal injection of atelocollagen in the latter half of the 1980s [116] and used the type I method [117] or AA [118] and a combination of these two methods [119], between 1990 and 2001. The numbers of patients treated with each approach are shown in the bottom four rows of Table 2.5. The patients included 31 males and 30 females, aged 19–84 years, with a mean age of 56.0 years.

Table 2.5 Vocal function after surgery reported in the literature. Mean values are cited

Operative method	Year reported	Authors	Number of subjects	Follow-up period	MPT(s)		MFR(mL/s)		Perceptual voice quality			
									Grade		Breathiness	
					Pre-op	Post-op	Pre-op	Post-op	Pre-op	Post-op	Pre-op	Post-op
Fat injection	1997	Shaw et al. [110]	11	1 year					4.7*	2.9*		
Fat injection	2002	McCulloch et al. [111]	8	52 days					2.1**	1.3**	1.4**	0.5**
Fascia injection	2002	Reijonen et al. [112]	14	13 m	5.8	11.4			3.3***	7.7***	3.1***	7.3***
Mixed fat and fascia injection	2009	Cheng et al. [113]	12	16.6 m	4.8	11.9			2.6**	1.3**	2.4**	0.9**
Insertion of rolled fascia	2006	Nishiyama et al. [45]	8	1 year	3.5	11.5	950	450				
Type I (silicon block)	1996	Lu et al. [114]	53	6 m	6.2	11.2	496	257				
Type I (Gore-Tex)	1998	McCulloch et al. [59]	14	6 m					2.3**	1.1**	2**	0.4**
Type I (silicon block)	2009	Suehiro et al. [115]	15	3 m	5.1	10.6	483	269				
Type I (Gore-Tex)	2009	Suehiro et al. [115]	15	3 m	6.7	12.6	550	221				
Arytenopexy + type I (Gore-Tex)	1999	Zeitels et al. [81]	10	<4 m	7	17.1	457	168				
AA + type I (Gore-Tex)	2000	McCulloch et al. [77]	19	>6 m	6.9	16.7			2.1**	0.8**	1.9**	0.2**
AA + type I (Gore-Tex)	2007	Tokashiki et al. [65]	12	6 m	2.8	19.6	898	150				
AA + collagen injection	2008	Kimura et al. [79]	40	>3 m	5	15	753	223				
AA + type I (silicon block)	2009	Mortensen et al. [78]	26	3 m	8.1	14.8	400	219				
Collagen injection [116]	The author's experience between Jan. 1986 and Apr. 2001		13	>3 m	5.8	7.0	324	226				
Type I (silicon block) [117]			12	>3 m	6.2	11.4	535	298				
AA alone [118]			15	>3 m	5.0	12.7	552	200				
AA + type I (silicon block) [119]			21	>3 m	3.7	10.4	525	207				

MPT maximum phonation time, *MFR* mean airflow rate

m months

Type I: Thyroplasty type I, *AA* Arytenoid adduction

*:1~5(1:normal, 5:severely disturbed)

**:0~3(0:normal, 3:severely disturbed)

***:0~10(0:severely disturbed, 10:normal)

A silicon block larger than that used in the original Isshiki method [52, 53] was employed for augmentation during application of the type I method. AA was performed under local anesthesia, and the type I method was added when AA alone did not adequately improve breathy dysphonia. All patients were followed up for at least 3 months.

Figures 2.7 and 2.8 show pre- and postoperative measurements of MPT and MFR, respectively, in patients treated using the type I method, via intracordal injection of atelocollagen, by AA, and with a combination of AA and the type I method. Intracordal injection of atelocollagen has not been performed since the 1990s, because the results were unsatisfactory. The author utilized autologous fat as an injection material to augment vocal fold performance in patients with mild breathy dysphonia or as a supplementary treatment after AA in patients with severe breathy dysphonia. Nearly half of all patients yielded MPT and MFR data after surgery that were less than 10 s and over 200 mL/s, respectively, regardless of the operative method chosen. Thus, the normal or near-normal voice of a patient with breathy dysphonia caused by UVFP is not always retrieved after framework surgery, including intracordal injection.

The number of patients with VFP associated with surgery has significantly increased since 1987 compared to the number over the prior 10 years. Phonosurgical procedures for treatment of paralytic dysphonia have developed rapidly over the past four decades. Postoperative voice is now definitely better than preoperative voice, but does not attain normal or even near-normal status. Previous reports on vocal outcomes after phonosurgical treatments refer to improvement in postopera-

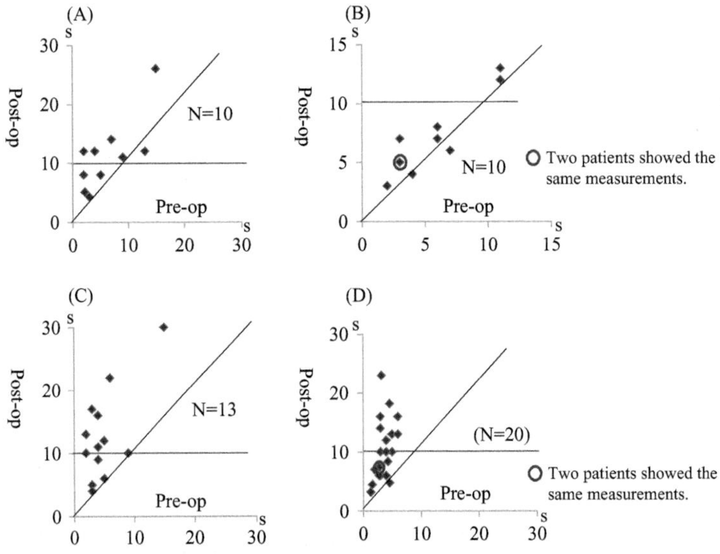

Fig. 2.7 Pre- and postoperative maximum phonation time after (**A**) thyroplasty type I (Type I), (**B**) collagen injection, (**C**) arytenoid adduction (AA), and a combination of (**D**) AA and Type I. The *blue line* indicates the lower limit of the normal range

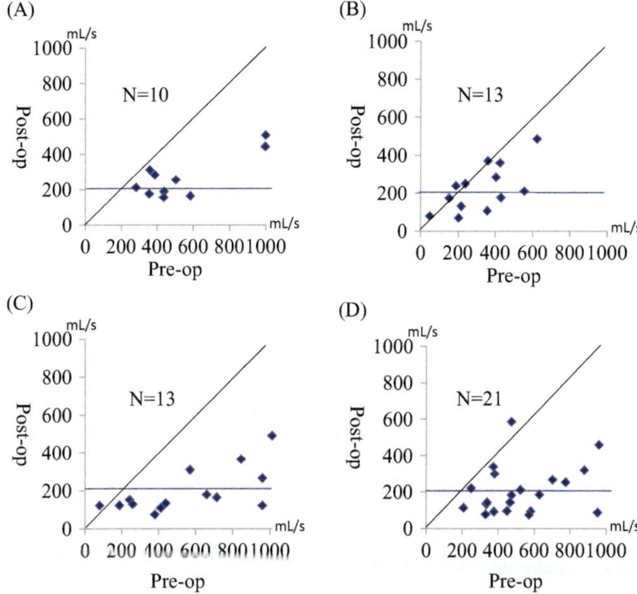

Fig. 2.8 Pre- and postoperative mean airflow rate after (**A**) thyroplasty type I (Type I), (**B**) colla-gen injection, (**C**) arytenoid adduction (AA), and a combination of (**D**) AA and Type I. The *blue line* indicates the upper limit of the normal range

tive compared to preoperative voice. Thus, postoperative voice is not compared to the voice of normal controls. Static correction of glottal configuration in terms of glottal closure and augmentation of the vocal fold is often insufficient to retrieve the vocal fold thickness, stiffness, and mass normally produced via TA muscle contrac-tion. Therefore, it appears to be essential to trigger TA muscle contraction, in addi-tion to median localization of the vocal fold, if a normal voice is to be recovered.

References

1. Smith E, Taylor M, Mendoza M, Barkmeier J, Lemke J, Hoffman H. Spasmodic dysphonia and vocal fold paralysis: outcomes of voice problems on work-related functioning. J Voice. 1998;12:223–32.
2. Benninger MS, Ahuja AS, Gardner G, Grywalski C. Assessing outcomes for dysphonic patients. J Voice. 1998;12:540–50.
3. Baba M, Natsugoe S, Shimada M, Nakano S, Noguchi Y, Kawachi K, Kusano C, Aikou T. Does hoarseness of voice from recurrent nerve paralysis after esophagectomy for carci-noma influence patient quality of life? J Am Coll Surg. 1999;188:231–6.
4. Fang TJ, Li HY, Glicklich RE, Chen YH, Wang PC, Chuang HF. Quality of life measures and predictors for adults with unilateral vocal cord paralysis. Laryngoscope. 2008;118:1837–41.

5. Bachor E, Bonkowsky V, Hacki T. Herpes simplex virus type I reactivation as a cause of a unilateral temporary paralysis of the vagus nerve. Eur Arch Otorhinolaryngol. 1996;253:297–300.

6. Amin MR, Koufman JA. Vagal neuropathy after upper respiratory infection: a viral etiology? Am J Otolaryngol. 2001;22:251–6.

7. Pinto JA, Pinto HCF, Ramalho JRO. Laryngeal herpes: a case report. J Voice. 2002;16:560–3.

8. Nakagawa H, Satoh M, Kusuyama T, Fukuda H, Ogawa K. Isolated vagus nerve paralysis caused by varicella zoster virus reactivation. Otolaryngol Head Neck Surg. 2005;133:460–1.

9. Chitose S, Umeno H, Hamakawa S, Nakashima T, Shoji H. Unilateral associated laryngeal paralysis due to varicella-zoster virus: virus antibody testing and videofluoroscopic findings. J Laryngol Otol. 2008;122:170–6.

10. Lin YY, Kao CH, Wang CH. Varicella zoster virus infection of the pharynx and larynx with multiple cranial neuropathies. Laryngoscope. 2011;121:1627–30.

11. Brunings W. Uber eine neue Behandlungsmethode der Rekurrenslamung. Verhandl ver Deutsch Laryngol. 1911;18:93–151.

12. Arnold GE. Alleviation of aphonia or dysphonia through intracordal injection of Teflon paste. Ann Otol Rhinol Laryngol. 1963;72:384–95.

13. Arnold GE. Further experiences with intracordal Teflon injection. Laryngoscope. 1964;74:802–15.

14. Ward PH. Use of injectable Teflon in otolaryngology. Arch Otolaryngol. 1968;87:637–43.

15. Donnellan WL, Gabriel W, Maurizi DG, et al. The use of silastic in the treatment of unilateral cord paralysis. An experimental study. Ann Otol Rhinol Laryngol. 1966;75:646–56.

16. Fukuda H. Vocal rehabilitation by silicon injection. Nippon Jibiinkouka Gakkai Kaiho. 1970;73:1506–26. (in Japanese)

17. Lewy RB. Teflon injection of the vocal cord: complications, errors, and precautions. Ann Otol Rhinol Laryngol. 1983;92:473–4.

18. Varvares MA, Montgomery WW, Hilman RE. Teflon granuloma of the larynx: etiology, pathophysiology, and management. Ann Otol Rhinol Laryngol. 1995;104:511–5.

19. Flint PW, Corio RL, Cummings CW. Comparison of soft tissue response in rabbits following laryngeal implantation with hydroxylapatite, silicone rubber, and Teflon. Ann Otol Rhinol Laryngol. 1997;106:399–407.

20. Andrews JM. Cellular behavior to injected silicone fluid: a preliminary report. Plast Reconstr Surg. 1966;38:581–3.

21. Tsuzuki T, Fukuda H, Fujioka T. Response of the human larynx to silicone. Am J Otolaryngol. 1991;12:288–91.

22. Ford CH, Bless DM. A preliminary study of injectable collagen in human vocal fold augmentation. Otolaryngol Head Neck Surg. 1986;94:104–22.

23. Mikaelian D, Lowry LD, Sataloff RT. Lipoinjection for unilateral vocal cord paralysis. Laryngoscope. 1991;101:465–9.

24. Laccourreye O, Papon JF, Kania R, et al. Intracordal injection of autologous fat in patients with unilateral laryngeal nerve paralysis: long-term results from the patient's perspective. Laryngoscope. 2003;113:541–5.

25. Rihkanen H. Vocal fold augmentation by injection of autologous fascia. Laryngoscope. 1998;108:51–4.

26. Duke SG, Salmon J, Blalock D, Postma GN, Koufman JA. Fascia augmentation of the vocal fold: graft yield in the canine and preliminary clinical experience. Laryngoscope. 2001;111:759–64.

27. Karpenko A, Dworkin J, Meleca R, et al. Cymetra injection for unilateral vocal fold paralysis. Ann Otol Rhinol Laryngol. 2003;112:927–34.

28. Milstein CF, Akst LM, Hicks D, Abelson TI, Strome M. Long-term effects of micronized AlloDerm injection for unilateral vocal fold paralysis. Laryngoscope. 2005;115:1691–6.

29. Belafsky PC, Postma GN. Vocal fold augmentation with calcium hydroxylapatite. Otolaryngol Head Neck Surg. 2004;131:351–4.
30. Carrol TL, Rosen CA. Long-term results of calcium hydroxylapatite for vocal fold augmentation. Laryngoscope. 2011;121:313–9.
31. Gillespie MB, Dozier TS, Day TA, Martin-Harris B, Nguyen SA. Effectiveness of hydroxylapatite paste in vocal rehabilitation. Ann Otol Rhinol Laryngol. 2009;118:546–51.
32. Finck C, Lefebvre P. Implantation of esterified hyaluronic acid in microdissected Reinke's space after vocal fold microsurgery: first clinical experiences. Laryngoscope. 2005;115:1841–7.
33. Upton DC, Johnson M, Zelazny SK, Dailey SH. Prospective evaluation of office-based injection laryngoplasty with hyaluronic acid gel. Ann Otol Rhinol Laryngol. 2013;122:541–6.
34. Sato K, Umeno H, Nakashima T. Autologous fat injection laryngopharyngoplasty for aspiration after vocal fold paralysis. Ann Otol Rhinol Laryngol. 2004;113:87–92.
35. Tamura E, Fukuda H, Tabata Y, Nishimura M. Use of the buccal fat pad for vocal cord augmentation. Acta Otolaryngol. 2008;128:219–24.
36. Tamura E, Fukuda H, Tabata Y. Adipose tissue formation in response to basic fibroblast growth factor. Acta Otolaryngol. 2007;127:1327–31.
37. Mikus JL, Koufman JA, Kilpatrick SE. Fate of liposuctioned and purified autologous fat injections in the canine vocal fold. Laryngoscope. 1995;105:17–22.
38. Bauer CA, Valentino J, Hoffman HT. Long-term result of vocal cord augmentation with autogenous fat. Ann Otol Rhinol Laryngol. 1995;104:871–4.
39. Cantarella G, Mazzola RF, Domenichini E, Arnone F, Maraschi B. Vocal fold augmentation by autologous fat injection with lipostructure procedure. Otolaryngol Head Neck Surg. 2005;132:239–43.
40. Tamura E, Okada S, Shibuya M, Iida M. Comparison of fat tissues used in intrcordal autologous fat injection. Acta Otolaryngol. 2010;130:405–9.
41. Tsunoda K, Takanosawa M, Niimi S. Autologous transplantation of fascia into the vocal fold: a new phonosurgical technique for glottal incompetence. Laryngoscope. 1999;109:504–8.
42. Tsunoda K, Niimi S. Autologous transplantation of fascia into the vocal fold. Laryngoscope. 2000;110:680–2.
43. Tsunoda K, Baer T, Niimi S. Autologous transplantation of fascia into the vocal fold: long-term results of a new phonosurgical technique for glottal incompetence. Laryngoscope. 2001;111:453–7.
44. Nishiyama K, Hirose H, Iguchi Y, Nagai H, Yamanaka J, Okamoto M. Autologous transplantation of fascia into the vocal fold as a treatment for recurrent nerve paralysis. Laryngoscope. 2002;112:1420–5.
45. Nishiyama K, Hirose H, Masaki T, Nagai H, Hashimoto D, Usui D, Yao K, Tsunoda K, Okamoto M. Long-term result of the new endoscopic vocal fold medialization surgical technique for laryngeal palsy. Laryngoscope. 2006;116:231–4.
46. Sulica L, Rosen CA, Postma GN, Simpson B, Amin M, Courey M, Merati A. Current practice in injection augmentation of the vocal folds: indications, treatment principles, techniques, and complications. Laryngoscope. 2010;120:319–25.
47. Payr E. Plastik am Schildknorpel zur Behebung der Folgen einseitiger Stimmbandlahmung. Dtsch Med Wochenschr. 1915;43:1265–70.
48. Meurmann Y. Operative mediofixation of the vocal cord in complete unilateral paralysis. Arch Otolaryngol. 1952;55:544–53.
49. Opheim O. Unilateral paralysis of the vocal cord. Acta Otolaryngol. 1955;45:226–30.
50. Sawashima M, Totsuka G, Kobayashi T, Hirose H. Surgery for hoarseness due to unilateral vocal cord paralysis. Arch Otolaryngol. 1968;87:289–94.
51. Bernstein L, Holt GP. Correction of vocal cord abduction in unilateral recurrent laryngeal nerve paralysis by transposition of the sternohyoid muscle. An experimental study in dogs. Laryngoscope. 1967;77:876–85.

52. Isshiki N, Morita H, Okamura H, Hiramoto M. Thyroplasty as a new phonosurgical technique. Acta Otolaryngol. 1974;78:451–7.
53. Isshiki N, Okamura H, Ishikawa T. Thyroplasty type I (lateral compression) for dysphonia due to vocal cord paralysis or atrophy. Acta Otolaryngol. 1975;80:465–73.
54. Carrau RL, Myers EN. Localization of true vocal cord for medialization thyroplasty. Laryngoscope. 1995;105:534–6.
55. Lee EC, Kuriloff DB. The pilot hole technique in type I thyroplasty. Laryngoscope. 1995;105:768–70.
56. Cummings CW, Purcell LL, Flint PW. Hydroxylapatite laryngeal implants for medialization: preliminary report. Ann Otol Rhinol Laryngol. 1993;102:843–51.
57. Montgomery WW, Montgomery SK. Montgomery thyroplasty implant system. Ann Otol Rhinol Laryngol. 1997;170(Suppl):1–16.
58. Friedrich G. Titanium vocal fold medialization implant: Introducing a novel implant system for external vocal fold medialization. Ann Otol Rhinol Laryngol. 1999;108:79–86.
59. McCulloch TM, Hoffman HT. Medialization laryngoplasty with expanded polytetrafluoroethylene. Surgical technique and preliminary results. Ann Otol Rhinol Laryngol. 1998;107:427–32.
60. Morrison LF. The "Reverse King operation". Ann Otol Rhinol Laryngol. 1948;57:945–56.
61. Montgomery WW. Cricoarytenoid arthrodesis. Ann Otol Rhinol Laryngol. 1966;75:380–91.
62. Isshiki N, Tanabe M, Sawada M. Arytenoid adduction for unilateral vocal cord paralysis. Arch Otolaryngol. 1978;104:555–8.
63. Iwamura S, Kurita N. A new arytenoid adduction technique for one-vocal-fold paralysis-a direct pull of the lateral cricoarytenoid muscle. Tokeibugeka. 1996;6:1–10. (in Japanese)
64. Sonoda S, Kataoka H, Inoue T. Traction of lateral cricoarytenoid muscle for unilateral vocal fold paralysis: comparison with Isshiki's original technique of arytenoids adduction. Ann Otol Rhinol Laryngol. 2005;114:132–8.
65. Tokashiki R, Hiramatsu H, Tsukahara K, Kanebayashi H, Nakamura M, Motohashi R, Yamada T, Suzuki M. A "fenestration approach" for arytenoid adduction through the thyroid ala combined with type I thyroplasty. Laryngoscope. 2007;117:1882–92.
66. Maragos NE. The posterior thyroplasty window: anatomical considerations. Laryngoscope. 1999;109:1228–31.
67. Su CY, Lui CC, Lin HC, Chiu JF, Cheng CA. A new paramedian approach to arytenoid adduction and strap muscle transposition for vocal fold medialization. Laryngoscope. 2002;112:342–50.
68. Slavit DH, Maragos NE. Physiologic assessment of arytenoid adduction. Ann Otol Rhinol Laryngol. 1992;101:321–7.
69. Su CY, Tsai SS, Chuang HCC, Chiu JF. Functional significance of arytenoid adduction with the suture attaching to cricoid cartilage versus to thyroid cartilage for unilateral paralytic dysphonia. Laryngoscope. 2005;115:1752–9.
70. Woodson GE, Picerno R, Yeung D, Hengesteg A. Arytenoid adduction: controlling vertical position. Ann Otol Rhinol Laryngol. 2000;109:360–4.
71. Rosen CA. Complications of phonosurgery: results of a national survey. Laryngoscope. 1998;108:1697–703.
72. Weinman EC, Maragos NE. Airway compromise in thyroplastic surgery. Laryngoscope. 2000;110:1082–5.
73. Abraham MT, Gonen M, Kraus DH. Complications of type I thyroplasty and arytenoids adduction. Laryngoscope. 2001;111:1322–9.
74. Maragos N. Pyriform sinus mucosa stabilization for prevention of postoperative airway obstruction in arytenoids adduction. Ann Otol Rhinol Laryngol. 2006;115:171–4.
75. Yumoto E, Nakano K, Oyamada Y, Hyodo M, Kobayashi J, Sanuki T. Laryngeal framework surgery for patients with unilateral vocal fold paralysis–present status and issues for future development. Tokeibugeka. 2001;11:83–9. (in Japanese)
76. Kraus DH, Orlikoff RF, Rizk SS, Rosenberg DB. Arytenoid adduction as an adjunct to type I thyroplasty for unilateral vocal cord paralysis. Head Neck. 1999;21:52–9.

77. McCulloch TM, Hoffman HT, Andrews BT, Karnell MP. Arytenoid adduction combined with Gore-tex medialization thyroplasty. Laryngoscope. 2000;110:1306–11.

78. Mortensen M, Carroll L, Woo P. Arytenoid adduction with medialization laryngoplasty versus injection or medialization laryngoplasty: the role of the arytenoidopexy. Laryngoscope. 2009;119:827–31.

79. Kimura M, Nito T, Imagawa H, Tayama N, Chan RW. Collagen injection as a supplement to arytenoid adduction for vocal fold paralysis. Ann Otol Rhinol Laryngol. 2008;117:430–6.

80. Zeitels SM, Hochman IH, Hillman RE. Adduction arytenopexy: a new procedure for paralytic dysphonia with implications for implant medialization. Ann Otol Rhinol Laryngol. 1998;107 Suppl 173:2–24.

81. Zeitels SM, Mauri M, Dailey SH. Adduction arytenopexy for vocal fold paralysis: indications and technique. J Laryngol Otol. 2004;118:508–16.

82. Zeitels SM, Hillman RE, Desloge RB, Bunting GA. Cricothyroid subluxation: a new innovation for enhancing the voice with laryngoplastic phonosurgery. Ann Otol Rhinol Laryngol. 1999;108:1126–31.

83. Haji T, Omori K, Mori K, Kojima H, Taira T, Isshiki N. Phonation after thyroplasty and arytenoid adduction. Pract Otorhinolaryngol. 1990;83:915–22. (in Japanese)

84. Isshiki N. Phonosurgery: theory and practice. Tokyo: Springer; 1989.

85. Nonomura M, Kojima H, Omori K, Kanaji M, Honjo I, Nakamura T, Shimizu Y. Remobilization of paralyzed vocal cord by anticus-lateralis muscle suturing. Arch Otolaryngol Head Neck Surg. 1993;119:498–503.

86. Nonomura M, Kojima H, Omori K, Ishijima K, Hirano S, Hopnjo I. Dynamic reconstruction for unilateral recurrent laryngeal nerve paralysis: clinical application of anticus-lateralis muscle suturing. Pract Otorhinolaryngol. 1992;85:1095–100.

87. Miyauchi A, Matsusaka K, Kihara M, Matsuzuka F, Hirai K, Yokozawa T, Kobayashi A, Kuma K. The role of ansa-to-recurrent laryngeal nerve anastomosis in operations for thyroid cancer. Eur J Surg. 1998;164:927–33.

88. Miyauchi A, Inoue H, Tomoda C, Fukushima M, Kihara M, Higashiyama T, Takamura Y, Ito Y, Kobayashi K, Miya A. Improvement in phonation after reconstruction of the recurrent laryngeal nerve in patients with thyroid cancer invading the nerve. Surgery. 2009;146:1056–62.

89. Yumoto E, Sanuki T, Kumai Y. Immediate recurrent laryngeal nerve reconstruction and vocal outcome. Laryngoscope. 2006;116:1657–61.

90. Sanuki T, Yumoto E, Minoda R, Kodama N. The role of immediate recurrent laryngeal nerve reconstruction for thyroid cancer surgery. J Oncol. 2010;846235.

91. Yumoto E, Gould J, Baer T. Harmonics-to-noise ratio as an index of the degree of hoarseness. J Acoust Soc Am. 1982;71:1544–50.

92. Tanaka S, Asato T, Hiratsuka Y. Nerve-muscle transplantation to the paraglottic space after resection of recurrent laryngeal nerve. Laryngoscope. 2004;114:1118–22.

93. Tucker HM. Reinnervation of the unilaterally paralyzed larynx. Ann Otol Rhinol Laryngol. 1977;86:789–94.

94. Tucker HM, Rusnov M. Laryngeal reinnervation for unilateral vocal cord paralysis: longterm results. Ann Otol Rhinol Laryngol. 1981;90:457–9.

95. Tucker HM. Combined laryngeal framework medicalization and reinnervation for unilateral vocal fold paralysis. Ann Otol Rhinol Laryngol. 1990;99:778–81.

96. Tucker HM. Combined surgical medicalization and nerve-muscle pedicle reinnervation for unilateral vocal fold paralysis: improved functional results and prevention of long-term deterioration of voice. J Voice. 1997;11:474–8.

97. Tucker HM. Long-term preservation of voice improvement following surgical medicalization and reinnervation for unilateral vocal fold paralysis. J Voice. 1999;13:251–6.

98. May M, Beery Q. Muscle-nerve pedicle laryngeal reinnervation. Laryngoscope. 1986;96:1196–200.

99. Maronian N, Waugh P, Robinson L, Hillel A. Electromyographic findings in recurrent laryngeal nerve reinnervation. Ann Otol Rhinol Laryngol. 2003;112:314–23.

100. Crumley RL, Izdebski K. Voice quality following laryngeal reinnervation by ansa hypoglossi transfer. Laryngoscope. 1986;96:611–6.
101. Crumley RL, Izdebski K, McMicken B. Nerve transfer versus Teflon injection for vocal cord paralysis: a comparison. Laryngoscope. 1988;98:1200–4.
102. Crumley RL. Update: ansa cervicalis to recurrent laryngeal nerve anastomosis for unilateral laryngeal paralysis. Laryngoscope. 1991;101:384–8.
103. Lorenz RR, Esclamado RM, Teker AM, Strome M, Scharpf J, Hicks D, Milstein C, Lee WT. Ansa cervicalis-to-recurrent laryngeal nerve anastomosis for unilateral vocal fold paralysis: experience of a single institution. Ann Otol Rhinol Laryngol. 2008;117:40–5.
104. Olson DL, Goding GS, Michael DD. Acoustic and perceptual evaluation of laryngeal reinnervation by ansa cervicalis transfer. Laryngoscope. 1998;108:1767–72.
105. Paniello RC. Laryngeal reinnervation with the hypoglossal nerve: II. Clinical evaluation and early patient experience. Laryngoscope. 2000;110:739–48.
106. Su WF, Hsu YD, Chen HC, Sheng H. Laryngeal reinnervation by ansa cervicalis nerve implantation for unilateral vocal cord paralysis in humans. J Am Coll Surg. 2007;204:64–72.
107. Paniello RC, Edgar JD, Kallogjeri D, Piccirillo JF. Medialization versus reinnervation for unilateral vocal fold paralysis: a multicenter randomized clinical trial. Laryngoscope. 2011;121:2172–9.
108. Chhetri DK, Gerratt BR, Kreinman J, Berke GS. Combined arytenoid adduction and laryngeal reinnervation in the treatment of vocal fold paralysis. Laryngoscope. 1999;109:1928–36.
109. Hassan MM, Yumoto E, Kumai Y, Sanuki T, Kodama N. Vocal outcome after arytenoid adduction and ansa cervicalis transfer. Aech Otolaryngol Head Neck Surg. 2012;138:60–5.
110. Shaw GY, Szewczyk MA, Searle J, Woodroof J. Autologous fat injection into the vocal folds: technical considerations and long-term follow-up. Laryngoscope. 1997;107:177–86.
111. McCulloch TM, Andrews BT, Hoffman HT, Graham SM, Karnell MP, Minnick C. Long-term follow-up of fat injection laryngoplasty for unilateral vocal cord paralysis. Laryngoscope. 2002;112:1235–8.
112. Reijonen P, Lehikoinen-Sodeerlund S, Rihkanen H. Results of fascial augmentation in unilateral vocal fold paralysis. Ann Otol Rhinol Laryngol. 2002;111:523–9.
113. Cheng Y, Li Z, Huang J, Xue F, Jiang M, Wu K, Wang Q. Combination of autologous fascia lata and fat injection into the vocal fold via the cricothyroid gap for unilateral vocal fold paralysis. Arch Otolaryngol Head Neck Surg. 2009;135:759–63.
114. Lu FL, Casiano RR, Lundy DS, Xue JW. Longitudinal evaluation of vocal function after thyroplasty type I in the treatment of unilateral vocal paralysis. Laryngoscope. 1996;106:573–7.
115. Suehiro A, Hirano M, Kishimoto Y, Tanaka S, Ford CN. Comparative study of vocal outcomes with silicone versus Gore-tex thyroplasty. Ann Otol Rhinol Laryngol. 2009;118:405–8.
116. Yumoto E, Okamoto K, Kawamura Y, Okamura H. Injection of atelocollagen to augment the paralyzed vocal fold. J Jpn Bronchoesophagol Soc. 1988;39:271–4. (in Japanese)
117. Yumoto E, Kadota Y. Thyroplasty type I as the treatment of hoarseness due to unilateral recurrent laryngeal nerve palsy. J Jpn Soc Head Neck Surg. 1993;3:161–7. (in Japanese)
118. Hyodo M, Yumoto E, Mori T, Kadota Y. Postoperative evaluation after arytenoid adduction. Practica Oto-Rhino-Laryngol. 1997;90:1129–34. (in Japanese)
119. Yumoto E, Oyamada Y, Goto H. Recent modifications in arytenoid adduction combined with type I thyroplasty. Larynx Jpn. 2003;15:78–83. (in Japanese)

Chapter 3
Denervation and Reinnervation of the Thyroarytenoid Muscle

Abstract The detailed effects of denervation on the intrinsic laryngeal muscles of rats were investigated. After denervation, the entire thyroarytenoid (TA) muscle and individual muscle fibers thereof gradually reduced in size over the next 10 weeks, but unlike muscles of the extremities, the dimensions then remained unchanged to 58 weeks of observation. Although nerve terminals disappeared within 24 h of nerve transection, approximately 70 % of the acetylcholine receptors (AchRs) were preserved at 10 weeks post-denervation. Subsequently, AchR numbers gradually decreased to 35 % of the initial value by 58 weeks after denervation. Nerve–muscle pedicle (NMP) flap implantation into the denervated TA muscle facilitated recovery of bulk muscle size, individual muscle fibers, neuromuscular junctions (NMJs), and function as reflected by evoked electromyography (EMG) testing. Such positive effects were noted even when the NMP procedure was performed 48 weeks post-injury, although treatment effects were less prominent as the time to treatment became extended. The NMP method also yielded favorable results in aged rats and animals in which the TA muscle became partially reinnervated after nerve injury.

Keywords Denervation • Reinnervation • Nerve–muscle pedicle flap • Muscle atrophy • Neuromuscular junction

3.1 Historical Review

3.1.1 Histological Changes in the Laryngeal Muscles After Denervation

Denervation of skeletal muscle decreases the mean cross-sectional areas of individual muscle fibers and reduces muscle size because of degradation, reduced protein synthesis, and apoptosis of muscle fibers [1]. Similar atrophic changes are also evident in the intrinsic laryngeal muscles, although they are not identical to changes in limb muscles. For example, 10 months after denervation, the rat soleus muscle decreased to 3 % of the muscle size on the normally innervated side, and few muscle

© Springer Japan 2015

E. Yumoto, *Pathophysiology and Surgical Treatment of Unilateral Vocal Fold Paralysis*, DOI 10.1007/978-4-431-55354-0_3

fibers with transverse striations were evident [2]. Furthermore, prolonged denervation (for up to 7 months) was accompanied by a pronounced decline in the number of myonuclei per muscle fiber in the rat extensor digitorum longus muscle [3]. However, atrophic changes in laryngeal muscles after denervation are considered to be less severe. Shindo et al. [4] explored the changes in canine laryngeal muscles after excision of a segment of the recurrent laryngeal nerve (RLN). The muscles initially underwent atrophy and fibrosis over the next 3 months, after which time partial reinnervation was noted as exemplified by the presence of hypertrophic muscle fibers and scattered areas of atrophy at 9 months. In the interval between 4 and 9 months, vocal fold movement was noted when the severed cranial end of the RLN was stimulated. It was believed that the reinnervation was attributable to regeneration of RLN nerve fibers. Shinners et al. [5] sectioned the RLN of rabbits and found that the number of bromodeoxyuridine (BrdU)-positive myonuclei in laryngeal muscles increased 1 week after denervation. In addition, the level of neonatal myosin heavy chain (MyHC) expression significantly increased until 24 weeks. It was suggested that these observations reflected an increase in satellite cell numbers, contributing to the ability of the laryngeal muscles to survive for extended periods following interruption of the nerve supply.

The process of degeneration has been examined at the neuromuscular junction (NMJ) level in muscles of the trunk and limbs. Winlow and Usherwood [6] reported that motor axon terminals disappeared 26 h after denervation of the mouse phrenic nerve. The number of AchRs in the soleus muscle of adult rats remained normal at 18 days but then fell to 54 % and 35 % of the initial value by 33 and 57 days, respectively. Thus, AchRs in NMJs persisted longer than motor axon terminals [7, 8].

3.1.2 Role of Basic Fibroblast Growth Factor in the Nucleus Ambiguus

The cell bodies of motor fibers innervating the intrinsic laryngeal muscles are located in the nucleus ambiguus (NA) [9–11]. Komori et al. [12] explored regeneration of motor fibers after RLN injury accompanied by administration of nerve growth factor, ciliary neurotrophic factor, or basic fibroblast growth factor (bFGF) at the site of injury and found that bFGF afforded the greatest protective effects in terms of regeneration of myelinated fibers. Moreover, bFGF prevented a decrease in the size of NA motor neurons that was noted in the controls. Sanuki et al. [13] measured bFGF expression levels in the NA after infliction of three different types of nerve injury on adult rats, which included nerve crush (Group A of Fig. 3.1; [Sunderland Grade II injury [14]]; Fig. 3.2) and nerve transection (Grade V injury, Fig. 3.2) without and with placement of caps on the nerve stumps to prevent regeneration (Groups B and C, respectively, of Fig. 3.1). The bFGF level in the NA of Group A was maximal 7 days after injury, whereas that of Group B peaked

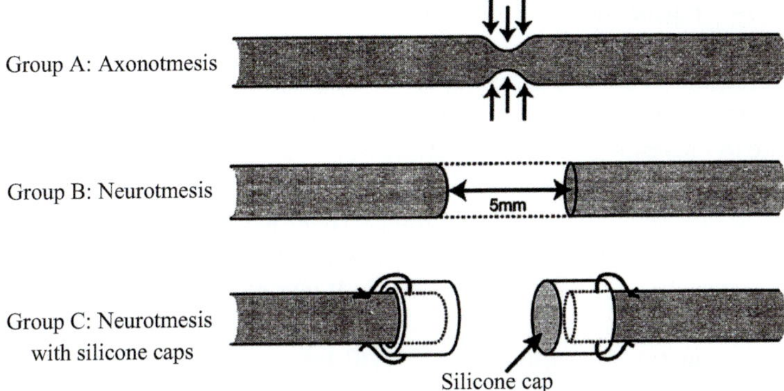

Fig. 3.1 Three different nerve injury models: group A, axonotmesis; group B, neurotmesis; and group C, neurotmesis featuring the use of silicone caps covering the severed ends of the recurrent laryngeal nerve (Citation: Ref. [14])

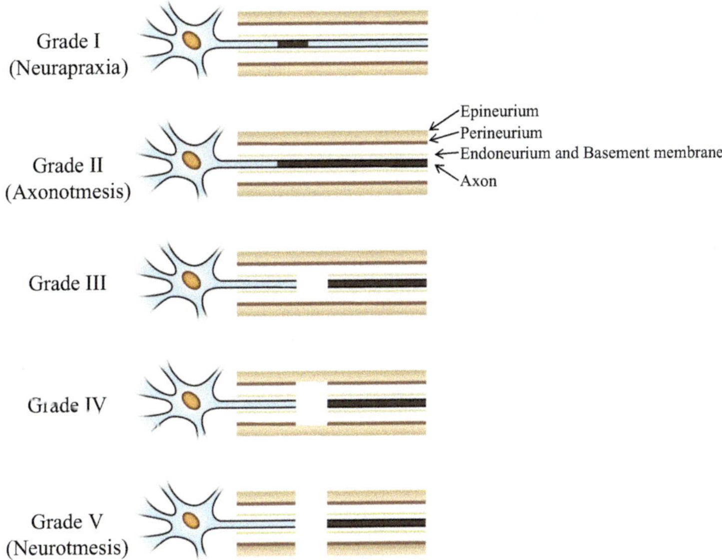

Fig. 3.2 Classification of peripheral nerve injuries according to Sunderland [14]. Grade I injury is sustained when conduction along the axon is interrupted at the site of injury, but no break in the continuity of structures comprising the nerve trunk is evident. Grade II injury is a situation in which the axon is severed, or the axonal mechanisms are so disorganized that the axon fails to survive below the level of the injury. Grade III injury is caused by more severe trauma, which, in addition to causing axonal disintegration and Wallerian degeneration, disorganizes the internal structure of the funiculi. Grade IV injury involves the entire funiculus; all bundles are so breached and disorganized that they are no longer sharply demarcated from the epineurium. Continuity of the nerve trunk is preserved, but the involved segment is ultimately converted into a tangled mass of connective tissue, Schwann cells, and regenerating axons. Grade V injury implies loss of continuity of the nerve trunk, associated with complete loss of motor, sensory, and sympathetic functions in the autonomous distribution region of the severed nerve

on day 14. Furthermore, Group B animals exhibited significantly greater immunoreactivity for and a longer duration of bFGF than those in Group A. However, the bFGF expression level in Group C was significantly lower than that in Groups A and B. It was concluded that endogenous bFGF in the NA might contribute to prevention of neuronal death induced by peripheral nerve injury and that blockage of axonal regeneration might suppress such bFGF production. Huber et al. [15] found that the level of messenger RNA (mRNA) encoding bFGF was higher in the hypoglossal nucleus following hypoglossal nerve injury caused by nerve transection rather than nerve crush. It was also found that local administration of bFGF at the site of nerve injury or at the NA prevented neuronal death after nerve transection. Fujimoto et al. [16] found that regenerating axons and Schwann cells promoted local bFGF production at the site of injury. Thus, blockage of axonal flow suppressed bFGF expression in the NA and may negatively affect neuronal survival in general.

3.1.3   Atrophic Changes in Laryngeal Muscle Fibers After Denervation

In general, striated muscles exhibit rapid atrophic changes after denervation [3, 17]. For example, Viguie et al. [3] reported that 2 months after denervation, the weight and contractile force of the rat extensor digitorum longus muscle fell to 31 % and 2 % of preinjury values, respectively. Kobayashi et al. [17] used a rat hind limb model to measure the extent of neuromuscular recovery at different times after nerve reconstruction. Although excellent axonal regeneration was noted irrespective of the denervation period, profound decreases were evident in the recovery of both muscle mass and integrated motor function if reconstruction was delayed for more than 1 month post-injury. It was noted that the extent of progressive change was not proportional to the length of the denervation period, but rather, that significant and more discrete changes developed later than 1 month after denervation and these changes precluded full recovery of muscle mass. Such findings have created discussion on the optimal timing and efficacy of reinnervation procedures used to treat chronic vocal fold paralysis.

Johns et al. [18] measured the isometric contraction force and the mass of the feline TA muscle 6 months after excision of a 3 cm long segment of the RLN and the external branch of the SLN. Isometric force and muscle mass decreased to 93 % and 85 %, respectively, compared to sham-treated animals, but no significant difference in either parameter was evident when denervated and sham-treated animals were compared. Such results suggest that it is possible to restore functional innervation of the TA muscle when reinnervation surgery is performed, even months after primary injury. The cited authors hypothesized that misdirected random regeneration occurred after denervation and that such synkinetic reinnervation may be helpful in preservation of muscle fiber structure and contractile capacity.

3.1.4 Changes in the Human Laryngeal Muscles and the Cricoarytenoid Joint After Denervation

A few histological reports on denervated human laryngeal muscles have appeared. Kirchner reported interesting histological findings in two patients with UVFP caused by jugular foramen syndrome and mediastinal disease who died 6 years and 7 months after the onset of UVFP, respectively [19, 20]. TA and PCA muscles that had been denervated for 6 years had disappeared and were replaced by fibrous tissue [19]. However, the interarytenoid (IA) muscle did not exhibit atrophic changes because of dual innervation from both RLNs [21]. In the patient who had experienced 7 months of denervation, the TA and PCA muscles exhibited severe atrophic and fibrotic changes [20]. Gacek and Gacek [22] histopathologically studied ten human whole-organ laryngeal specimens with histories of long-standing paralysis (from 6 months to 17 years) to determine changes in laryngeal muscles. Muscle fibers were observed in the TA, LCA, and PCA muscles, although the muscles were atrophic in patients with unilateral paralysis. As described in Chap. 1, many animal experiments have confirmed that reinnervation of laryngeal muscles occurs after denervation of the RLN. Thus, it is considered that laryngeal muscles maintain their muscle fibers to a certain extent, thereby sustaining the capacity to accept regenerating nerve fibers and form neuromuscular junctions after injury to the RLN. More work on human larynges denervated for months or years is necessary to confirm this point.

Again, there have been only a few reports on changes in the cricoarytenoid (CA) joint after onset of VFP. Contracture of joint movement develops after paralysis of the extremities if no rehabilitative intervention is applied. However, Gacek and Gacek [22] found that the CA joint maintained a normal histological structure without fibrosis, osseous obliteration of joint space, or degeneration of the articular surface in ten paralyzed human larynges. Müller and Paulsen [23] performed laser arytenoidectomy on ten patients with bilateral VFP 6 weeks to 44 years in duration and histologically examined the joint surfaces of the arytenoid cartilage. In specimens from patients with paralysis 9 and 30 months in duration, changes in the superficial layer were evident with formation of chondrocyte clusters, a decrease in the total cell counts in the upper cartilage layer, and development of a clear demarcation line between that layer and underlying cartilage of normal appearance. Such specimens also exhibited roughness of the joint surface of the cartilage. One specimen from a patient with paralysis 30 years in duration exhibited a fibrous coating in certain areas that covered the underlying cartilage. Although clear structural changes were notable on the articular surface of the arytenoid cartilage, CA joint ankylosis was absent, even in a patient with paralysis 44 years in duration. The absence of such ankylosis was attributed to continuous passive movement of the joint during swallowing and small residual contractions of the laryngeal muscles, which may receive regenerating nerve fibers.

In summary, atrophic changes in laryngeal muscles develop after VFP onset, but the muscle fibers remain intact for a relatively long period of time. The time from onset of VFP to the disappearance of muscle fibers depends on the presence and extent of laryngeal muscle reinnervation. Furthermore, CA joint ankylosis does not develop, even many years after VFP onset. Thus, surgical treatments seeking to adduct the vocal fold and reinnervate the laryngeal muscles are feasible in patients with long-standing VFP. Further work is required to identify the optimal interval from onset of VFP to surgery.

3.1.5 Reinnervation of Denervated Muscle

Functionally efficient regeneration of nerve fibers can be expected after Grade I or II nerve injuries. However, when a nerve injury is worse than Grade III, axonal regeneration is complicated by disruption of the endoneurium and local fibrosis, and functional recovery is rarely expected as the extent of nerve injury increases. In addition, if a nerve is injured at a proximal level, apoptosis of the motor neuron may develop, thereby reducing the numbers of regenerating axons.

Clinical methods used to reinnervate a denervated muscle include direct suturing of the severed nerve ends, interposition of a portion of a foreign nerve between the transected nerve ends, and nerve transfer (Fig. 2.6, Chap. 2). Because the RLN consists of a single funiculus, nerve suturing is performed using the perineural suture technique. Interposition of a piece of foreign nerve is preferable when the gap between the cut ends is longer than 3–5 mm, because tension at the suture site often causes poor axonal regeneration if the suture ruptures unexpectedly and reduces blood flow. Nerve transfer is the method of choice when the cranial end of the nerve is unavailable for reconstruction. Foreign nerve fibers regenerate into the peripheral nerve and can produce neuromuscular junctions [24]. The ansa cervicalis nerve (ACN) is utilized for such a purpose, because that nerve is of a similar diameter to the RLN and is located in proximity to the latter nerve. In addition, the ACN consists principally of motor axons. Reconstruction of the RLN during tumor extirpation from the neck favorably affects vocal function, although vocal fold movement does not recover [25–28].

Any of the abovementioned three methods can be used when the peripheral end of the RLN is available for reconstruction. Figure 3.3 shows four different reinnervation methods applicable to the treatment of denervated muscle when the peripheral end of the nerve is unavailable for reconstruction. Experimentally, implantation of a foreign motor nerve into a denervated muscle (a nerve implant, NI) has been reported to produce new NMJs [29, 30]. In 2007, Su et al. [31] performed NI on the TA muscle of ten patients, using the ACN, to treat paralytic dysphonia and reported that eight patients exhibited improvements in voice quality at the 2-year follow-up. However, the absence of further positive reports on NI has discouraged clinical utilization of the method. Muscular neurotization is a phenomenon whereby one muscle innervates an adjacent denervated muscle via collateral nerve sprouts [32, 33]. Muscle–nerve–muscle (MNM) neurotization is defined as reinnervation of a denervated muscle via axons in a nerve graft that are induced to sprout from motor nerves within an innervated muscle. Reinnervation of the target muscle occurs via these axons. Using animal models, Hogikyan et al. [34] and Debnath et al. [35] histologically and electromyographically demonstrated reinnervation of denervated laryngeal muscles after MNM neurotization. However, neither muscular nor MNM neurotization has been clinically applied for laryngeal reinnervation. Previously, a nerve–muscle pedicle (NMP) flap was used to ameliorate inspiratory distress in patients with bilateral VFP via transfer of an intact nerve with a portion of the muscle supplied by that nerve [36]. This muscle fragment, together with the associated nerve pedicle, is sutured into the paralyzed muscle. Even a small muscle fraction contains a large number of cut nerve fibers, and every cut end branches and regenerates into the denervated muscle to form new NMJs (Fig. 3.4) [37]. Tucker [38, 39] and May and Beery [40] reported improvements in postoperative voice after NMP flap implantation into the TA and LCA muscles, respectively, but the method has not been widely accepted as a treatment for paralytic dysphonia because of the lack of further favorable reports.

Frey et al. [32] compared reinnervation efficiency using three different methods (direct suturing, NI, muscular neurotization) of the rectus femoris muscle of the rabbit and showed that both nerve suturing and NI were superior to muscular neurotization. Meikle studied the relative effectiveness of the NI and NMP flap methods using denervated strap muscles of a rabbit model and obtained similar effects using the two reinnervation methods [37]. The cited authors considered that a possible bar to successful reinnervation might arise when the original nerve supply was present

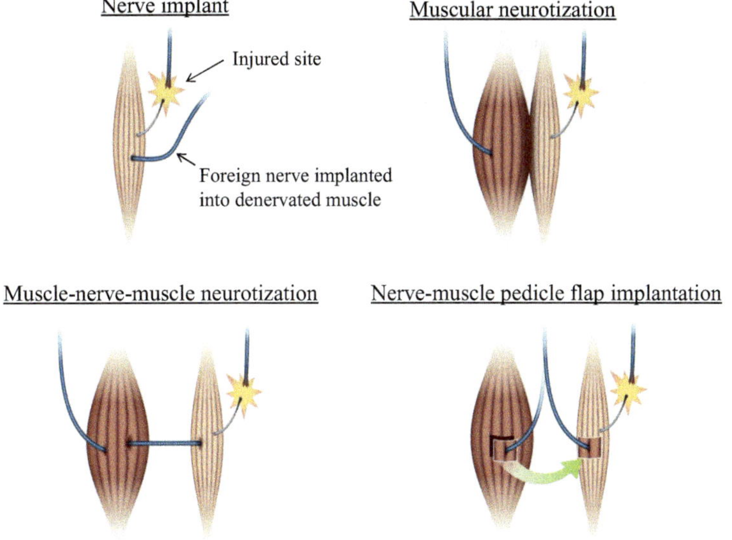

Fig. 3.3 Reinnervation methods for denervated muscle when the peripheral end of the nerve is unavailable for reconstruction; these are nerve implantation, muscular neurotization, muscle–nerve–muscle neurotization, and nerve–muscle pedicle (NMP) flap implantation

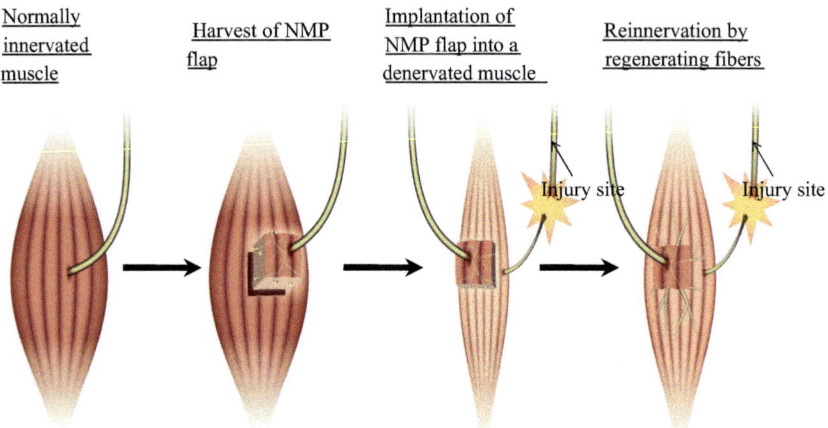

Fig. 3.4 Reinnervation of a denervated muscle after implantation of a nerve–muscle pedicle (*NMP*) flap

but nonfunctional, inhibiting development of newly implanted muscle. Zheng et al. [41] used electromyographic and histological techniques to compare the effects of nerve suturing, NI, and NMP implantation on reinnervation of the canine laryngeal adductor muscles. It was noted that nerve suturing was superior to NI and the use of the NMP technique and that little difference was evident between the outcomes of the latter two methods. In general, denervated muscle fibers can form NMJs at new sites during reinnervation [42]. However, the reinnervation process (growth of nerve fibers and formation of NMJs) may be negatively affected by subclinical regeneration of the RLN back to the laryngeal muscles, because NMJ formation in innervated muscle fibers, using foreign nerve fibers, is inhibited by continuation of the original local innervation [37]. Thus, Zheng et al. [41] suggested that the RLN should be severed prior to application of a reinnervation protocol. The present author explored the effect of NMP flap implantation into the denervated TA muscle of the rat and found that this effectively reduced atrophic changes in the TA muscle even in the presence of partial innervations thereof [43]. Details of this study will be described below, in Sect. 3.3.4.

3.2   Changes in the TA Muscle After Denervation

Injury to a peripheral nerve triggers degeneration and atrophy of muscle fibers and NMJs. Although such changes after muscle denervation have been investigated in the extremities [3, 44, 45], only a few studies on changes in laryngeal muscles after denervation have appeared. This section describes degenerative and atrophic changes in the TA muscle after denervation via transection of the rat RLN.

3.2.1   Short-Term Changes in Muscles

3.2.1.1   The Animal Model

Eight-week-old Wistar rats were anesthetized by intraperitoneal injection of ketamine (50 mg/kg) and xylazine (10 mg/kg). Under an operating microscope, the left RLN was exposed and resected at the level of the seventh tracheal ring, with removal of a 10 mm long segment. The distal end of the nerve was ligatured with 4-0 nylon and the proximal end embedded into the sternohyoid muscle to prevent contact between the two cut ends. The skin incision was closed, and the rats were allowed to recover in an approved animal care facility.

The animals were divided into eight groups defined by the length of the observation period after treatment: seven groups underwent left laryngeal nerve manipulation, and the final group was a non-treatment control group. Six animals in each group were killed by administration of an overdose of pentobarbital at 6, 12, 18, and 24 h and 2, 4, and 10 weeks after treatment. Larynges were isolated, frozen in liquid nitrogen, embedded in an OCT compound, and stored at −80 °C. Coronal sections (7 8 μm thick) of frozen larynges were prepared using a cryostat [46].

3.2.1.2   Areas of the Entire TA Muscle and Individual Muscle Fibers

To evaluate the areas of the entire TA muscle and those of individual muscle fibers, we examined sections within an area approximately 300 μm behind the front edge of the arytenoid cartilage; the sections were stained with hematoxylin and eosin. We matched sections of bilateral TA muscles using the contours of the arytenoid cartilages as guides and measured both TA muscle areas and those of individual muscle fibers (30–50) in three-to-five matched sections from each animal. We calculated the areas between the treated (left, T) and untreated (right, U) sides (deriving a T/U ratio) of the same section. In addition, in the six control animals, the entire muscle areas and those of individual TA muscle fibers were evaluated by comparing data from the left and right sides; the results are shown in Fig. 3.5. The unpaired Student's *t*-test was used to perform statistical analysis, and a difference was considered significant at a P value less than 0.05.

Figure 3.5 shows changes over time in total muscle area and that of individual muscle fibers in a coronal section of the TA muscle after transection of the left RLN. Figure 3.6 shows representative microscopic findings on the TA muscle (hematoxylin and eosin stained) 10 weeks after transection of the left RLN. At 24 h after treatment, neither the entire TA muscle nor that of individual muscle fibers differed significantly from those of the control. In contrast, both of these parameters decreased significantly by 2 weeks posttreatment (P<0.05), and at 10 weeks, the T/U ratios of the entire muscle area and that of the muscle fibers were 53.2±10.7 % and 55.5±6.8 %, respectively (control: 100 %) (P<0.01).

As mentioned in Sect. 3.1.3, the weight of the rat extensor digitorum longus muscle decreased to 31 % of the pretreatment value 2 months after denervation [3]. Thus, compared to muscles of the extremities, atrophic changes in the TA muscle after denervation develop gradually over 10 weeks in rats.

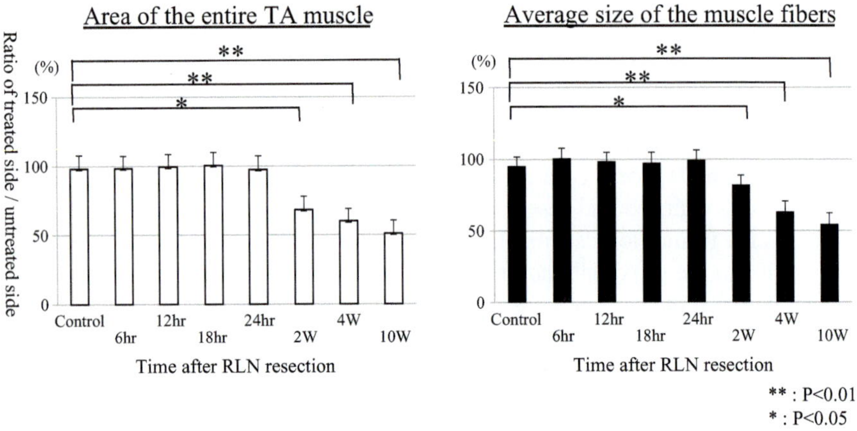

Fig. 3.5 Temporal changes in total muscle area (*left*) and that of individual muscle fibers (*right*) of the thyroarytenoid (*TA*) muscle after transection of the left recurrent laryngeal nerve (*RLN*). All data are presented as means ± SDs (Citation: Ref. [46])

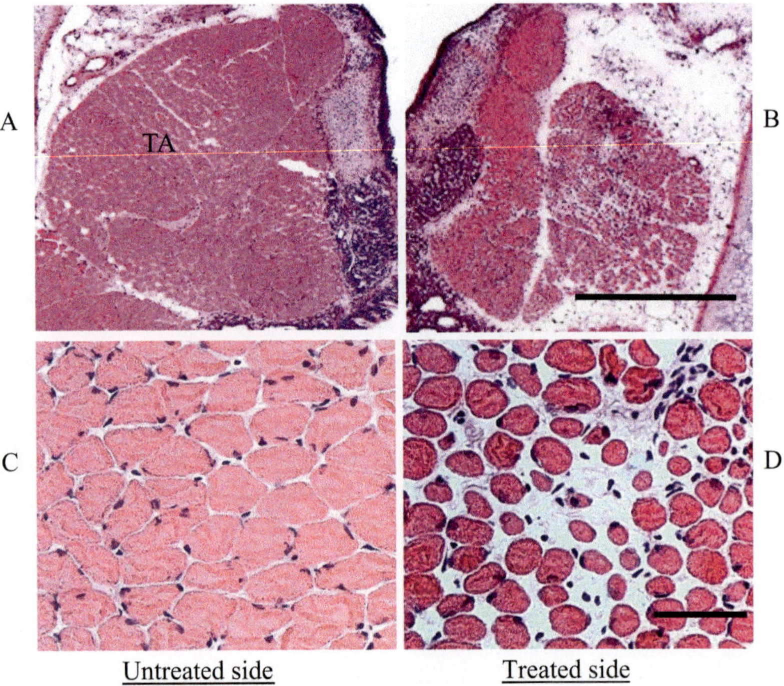

Fig. 3.6 Representative microscopic findings on the thyroarytenoid (*TA*) muscle (upon hematoxylin–eosin staining) 10 weeks after transection of the left recurrent laryngeal nerve. (**A, C**) the untreated right side and (**B, D**) the treated left side. Scale bars: **A** and **B** 1 mm; **C, D** 50 μm (Citation: Ref. [46])

3.2.1.3   The Neuromuscular Junction

We selected sections from the area embracing the middle one-third of the thyroid cartilage, because this region is rich in NMJs. An NMJ features pre- and postsynaptic structures, interrupted by a synaptic cleft (Fig. 3.7). Synaptophysin is a protein constituent of the presynaptic vesicle membrane [47], and thus, motor axon terminals can be histologically visualized via immunostaining for synaptophysin. Alphabungarotoxin (α-BTX) exhibits high affinity for the AchRs of skeletal muscle; therefore, motor endplates can be visualized using fluorescently labeled α-BTX [48]. The structures described above interact to form and maintain NMJs during denervation and reinnervation.

The number of synaptophysin-positive nerve terminals and α-BTX-positive AchRs in the entire TA muscle from the T (left) and U (right) sides of eight randomly selected sections from a single animal were counted. Next, the ratios of the numbers of synaptophysin-positive nerve terminals or α-BTX-positive AchRs on the T and U sides were determined, and T/U ratios were calculated. The ratios obtained from all 48 sections of each experimental group were averaged.

In the normal TA muscle, synaptophysin-immunoreactive sites and α-BTX-stained sites matched well. At 24 h, the number of α-BTX binding sites did not significantly differ between the two sides. However, the number of α-BTX binding sites decreased significantly ($P<0.05$) at 10 weeks posttreatment (to 70.5 ± 12.4 % that of the control) (Figs. 3.8 and 3.9). The number of nerve terminals decreased significantly ($P<0.01$) by 18 h (45.2 ± 6.8 %), and such terminals disappeared by 24 h posttreatment.

Such rapid degeneration of presynaptic nerve terminals after denervation of peripheral nerves has been studied [6]. On the other hand, AchRs persist for a

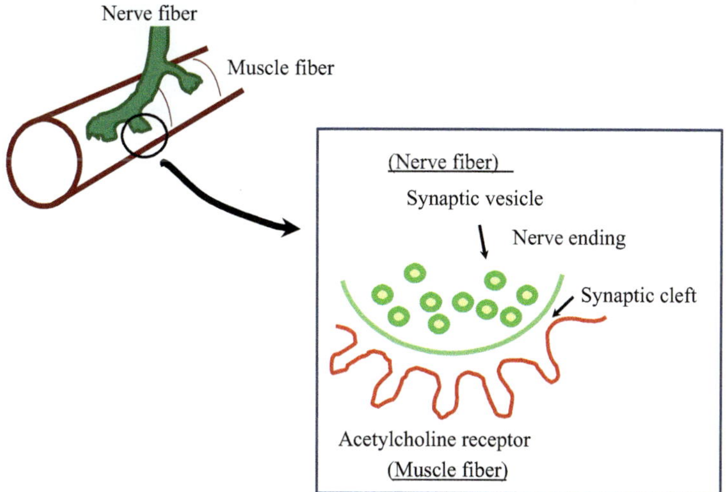

Fig. 3.7 Schematic drawing of the structure of the neuromuscular junction

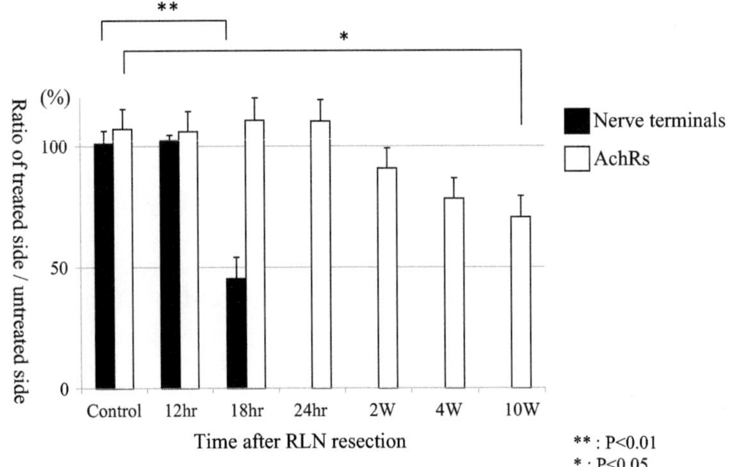

Fig. 3.8 Temporal changes in the numbers of nerve terminals (*black bars*) and acetylcholine receptors (*AchRs*) (*white bars*) in neuromuscular junctions of the thyroarytenoid muscle in a control group and in a group that underwent recurrent laryngeal nerve (*RLN*) transection. All data are presented as means ± SDs (Citation: Ref. [46])

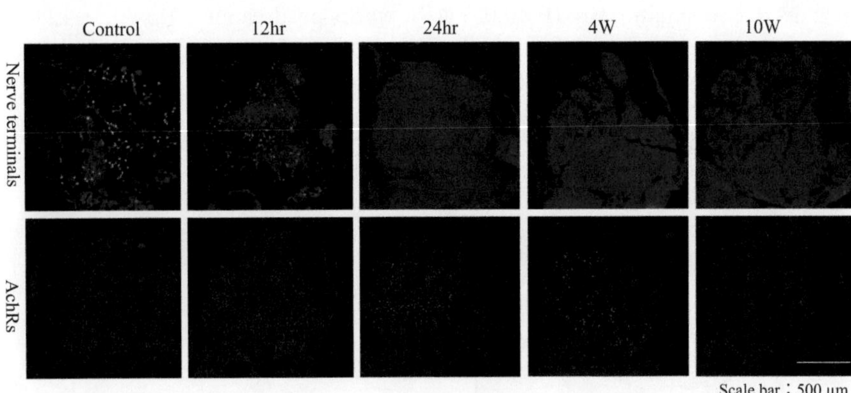

Fig. 3.9 Serial sections of the rat thyroarytenoid (*TA*) muscle from control animals and from test animals taken at 12 h, 24 h, 4 weeks, and 10 weeks after transection of the recurrent laryngeal nerve (*RLN*). Neuromuscular junctions (*NMJs*) are doubly stained with fluorescein isothiocyanate-labeled synaptophysin and rhodamine-labeled α-bungarotoxin (*BTX*) (Citation: Ref. [46])

relatively long period compared to nerve terminals [7, 8]. For example, the number of AchRs in the soleus muscle of the adult rat was normal to 18 days post-denervation and then fell by 65 % by 57 days [8]. We found no significant decrease in AchR numbers until 4 weeks after RLN transection, and even at 10 weeks, approximately 70 % of AchR reactivity was preserved. Thus, compared to the muscles of the extremities, AchR degradation in the TA muscle after denervation occurs gradually over 10 weeks in rats.

3.2.2 Long-Term Changes in the TA Muscle

Only a few studies have explored long-term muscle atrophy after denervation; this is an important question, because the presence of muscle fibers is a prerequisite for successful reinnervation. In addition, since AchRs are targeted by regenerating axon sprouts during reinnervation, muscle fibers must retain AchRs to accommodate the new connections. In theory, higher numbers of preserved AchRs should lead to more efficient reinnervation. In this section, local effects upon long-term denervation of the TA muscle of rats will be described. The method used was described in Sect. 3.2.1. Observations were made 10, 18, 26, 42, and 58 weeks after denervation, and each group contained six animals [49].

3.2.2.1   Areas of the Entire TA Muscle and Individual Muscle Fibers

The T/U ratios of the entire muscle area and individual muscle fibers fell significantly by 10 weeks post-denervation (P<0.01) compared to the control group; such changes were noted in all denervation groups. These two indices were relatively similar, regardless of the denervation period, ranging from 61.1 to 72.5 % and 45.0 to 51.9 %, respectively (Fig. 3.10). Atrophy of the TA muscle and proliferation of connective tissue around and between the fibers of that muscle were evident on the treated side (Fig. 3.11). Fibrotic connective tissue accounted for a more prominent decrease in individual muscle fibers than in the entire muscle bulk.

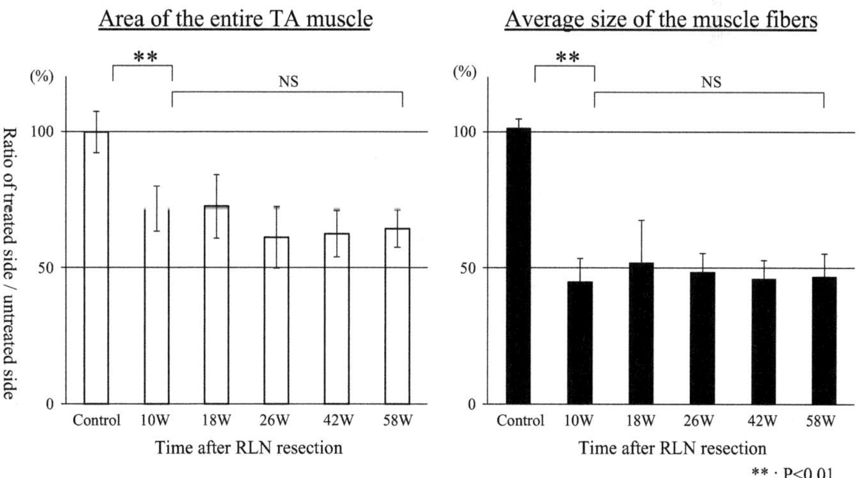

Fig. 3.10 Temporal changes in total muscle area and that of individual muscle fibers in coronal sections of the thyroarytenoid (*TA*) muscle prepared after transection of the left recurrent laryngeal nerve (*RLN*). All data are presented as means ± SDs (Citation: Ref. [49])

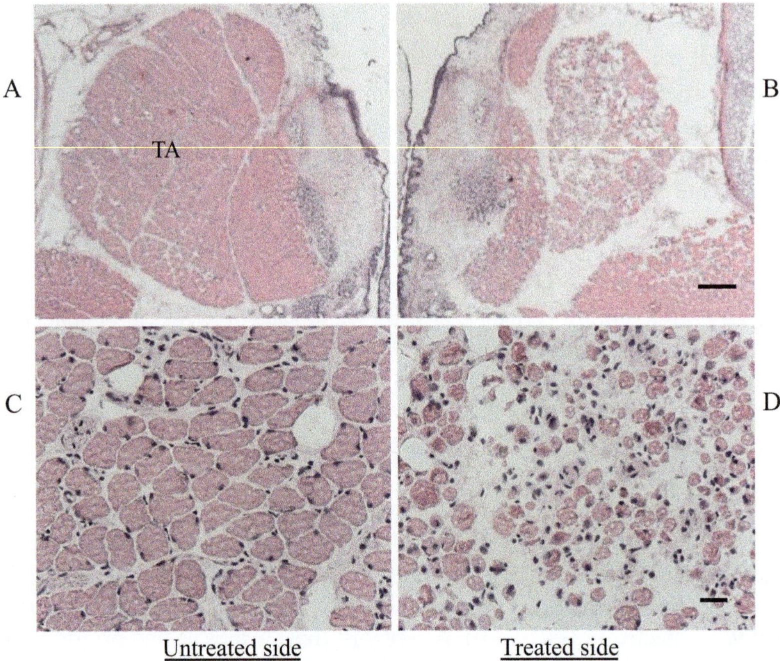

Fig. 3.11 Representative microscopic findings on the thyroarytenoid (*TA*) muscle (after hematoxylin–eosin staining) 58 weeks after transection of the left recurrent laryngeal nerve (*RLN*). (**A**, **C**) untreated *right side* and (**B**, **D**) treated *left side*. Scale bars: **A** and **B** 200 μm; **C** and **D** 20 μm (Citation: Ref. [49])

3.2.2.2   The Neuromuscular Junction

In our comprehensive study, we found that nerve terminals were not evident at the low magnification (50×) used in our short-term work, whereas such terminals were counted under a higher magnification (200×) in the long-term study. Thus, the numbers of nerve terminals evident 10 weeks after denervation were greater in the long-term study than in the short-term study. The T/U ratios of nerve terminals and AchRs were significantly lower in the denervation groups than in the control group. Both indices continued to fall after prolonged denervation, namely, at 10 and 58 weeks (being 26.3±4.1 % and 76.3±9.0 % at 10 weeks; 13.4±11.9 % and 35.3±20.2 % at 58 weeks) (Fig. 3.12). Furthermore, the number of synaptophysin-positive sites that also stained with α-BTX (i.e., AchRs) was compared to the number of total observable AchRs on the treated side. The ratios in the denervation groups were significantly smaller than that of the controls. However, the index values (which ranged from 30.3 to 35.6 %) did not differ significantly among the five denervation groups (Fig. 3.13). Figure 3.14 shows representative microscopic findings on the TA muscle, specifically stained for nerve terminals and AchRs at 10 and 58 weeks after RLN transection.

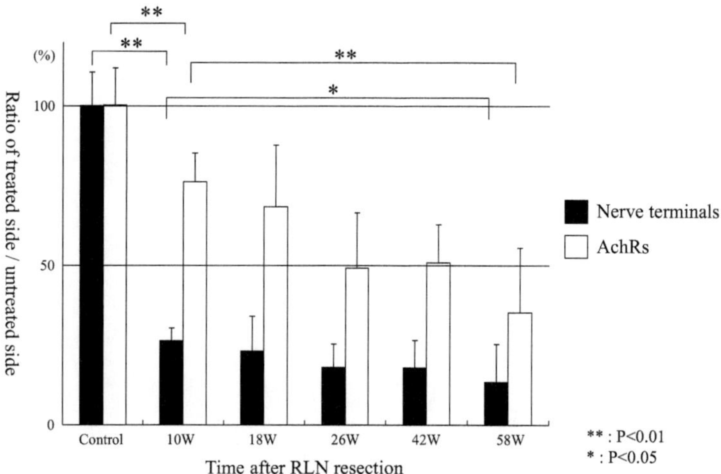

Fig. 3.12 Temporal changes in the numbers of nerve terminals (*black bars*) and acetylcholine receptors (*AchRs*) (*white bars*) in neuromuscular junctions of the thyroarytenoid muscle in a control group and after recurrent laryngeal nerve (*RLN*) transection. All data are presented as means ± SDs (Citation: Ref. [49])

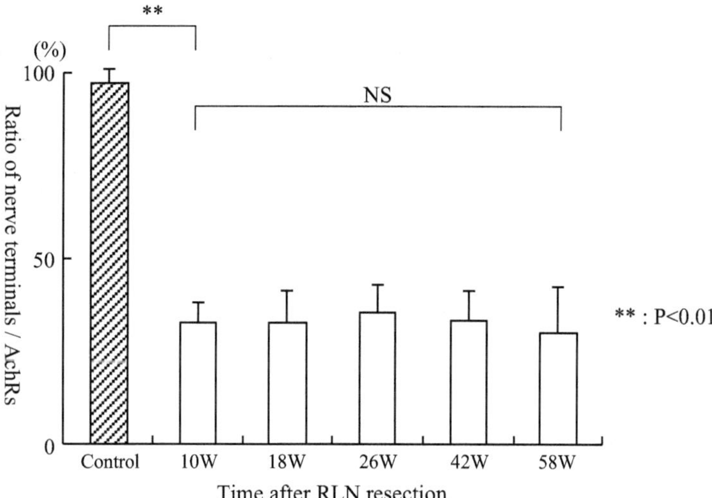

Fig. 3.13 Temporal changes in the ratios of the numbers of nerve terminals compared to those of acetylcholine receptors (*AchRs*) in the left thyroarytenoid (*TA*) muscle after left recurrent laryngeal nerve (*RLN*) resection. *Shaded bars*: untreated sides. All data are presented as means ± SDs (citation: Ref. [49])

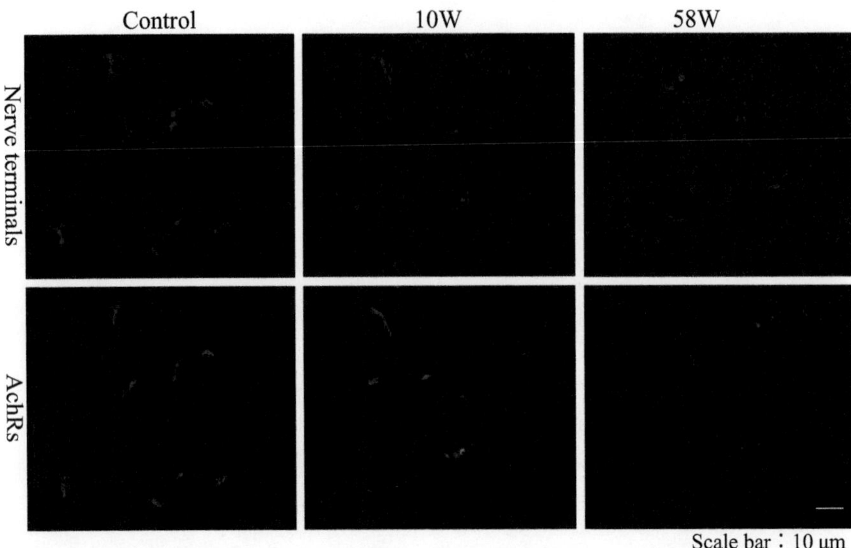

Fig. 3.14 Representative microscopic findings on the rat thyroarytenoid (*TA*) muscle in control animals and in test animals 10 and 58 weeks after transection of the recurrent laryngeal nerve (*RLN*). Neuromuscular junctions (*NMJs*) were doubly stained with fluorescein isothiocyanate-labeled synaptophysin and rhodamine-labeled α-bungarotoxin (*BTX*) (Citation: Ref. [49])

3.2.2.3 Discussion

Among the denervated groups, the average T/U ratios for the entire TA muscle area and that of individual muscle fibers did not significantly change from 10 to 58 weeks post-injury. Furthermore, the ratios of nerve terminal to AchR numbers did not vary at the different time points. However, although nerve terminals were present in the NMJs of all groups, the T/U ratios of nerve terminals and AchRs were significantly lower at 58 weeks than at 10 weeks.

We believe that a denervated TA muscle may be reinnervated by the original resected RLN [4, 18], autonomic nerves [50], superior laryngeal nerve [51], or other nerves. Such reinnervation may preserve muscle fibers both morphologically and functionally. Johns et al. [18] reported that the maximal isometric force of the feline TA muscle did not change for 6 months after RLN resection. It was hypothesized that the contractile force was preserved via spontaneous reinnervation of the resected RLN. In contrast, in the rat gastrocnemius muscle, the contractile force was significantly impaired 1 month post-injury [17]. Other studies on laryngeal muscles revealed that AchRs were preserved for several weeks after denervation in rats. However, long-term observations over 58 weeks showed that the number of AchRs decreased gradually after denervation. Thus, the ability of a denervated TA muscle to receive regenerating nerve axons may gradually decline, and a reinnervated muscle may fail to recover sufficient function after prolonged denervation. Because the life expectancy of rats is 2.5–3 years, the presence of AchRs and functional muscle fibers 58 weeks after denervation in this animal model suggests that human laryngeal muscles might retain the ability to accommodate regenerating axons with formation of functional connections for several years after VFP onset.

3.3   Nerve–Muscle Pedicle (NMP) Flap Implantation into the TA Muscle

Implantation of an NMP flap using the ACN has been clinically applied to reinnervate PCA and TA muscles when the peripheral end of the RLN could not be located because of severe cicatricial changes [38, 39, 52]. However, the question of whether NMP flap implantation can be used to reinnervate denervated laryngeal muscles remains controversial, even in the experimental context. Tucker's group [53, 54] reported that reinnervation of denervated PCA muscles via NMP flap implantation was effective. Anonsen et al. [55] performed strap muscle NMP transfer to the contralateral denervated strap muscle of rabbits and demonstrated functional reinnervation both electromyographically and histochemically. Fata et al. [56] examined the outcomes of ansa cervicalis NMP flap implantation into denervated feline PCA muscle using a glycogen depletion method and demonstrated successful reinnervation. However, Rice et al. [57] and Crumley [58] implanted NMP flaps into the PCA muscles of cats and dogs and found no evidence of reinnervation upon histological and electromyographic examination. The ineffectiveness of NMP flap transfer was attributed to development of local fibrosis that interfered with the growth of sprouting nerve fibers toward target muscle fibers.

In this section, the outcomes of NMP flap implantation immediately after denervation of the rat TA muscle will be described. We explore three specific issues that were not evaluated in previous studies; these are modulation of atrophic processes within a denervated TA muscle, re-formation of NMJs, and changes in myosin heavy chain (MyHC) composition of the muscle.

3.3.1   Immediate Implantation

The rat RLN was transected on the left side and managed as described in Sect. 3.2.1.1 (denervation-alone animals are referred to as the DNV group). Subsequently, other animals with transected left RLNs underwent NMP implantation. Under an operating microscope, the ACN was identified and followed until the nerve entered the sternohyoid (SH) muscle. The ACN was electrically stimulated to confirm that the SH muscle was innervated by that ACN. A branch of the ACN, together with a 0.5×0.5×0.5-mm piece of SH muscle, was harvested and implanted into the TA muscle through a small window constructed in the thyroid cartilage. The NMP flap was firmly sutured to the surface of the TA muscle using 10-0 nylon (Fig. 3.15). After completion of this procedure, the skin incision was closed, and all rats were

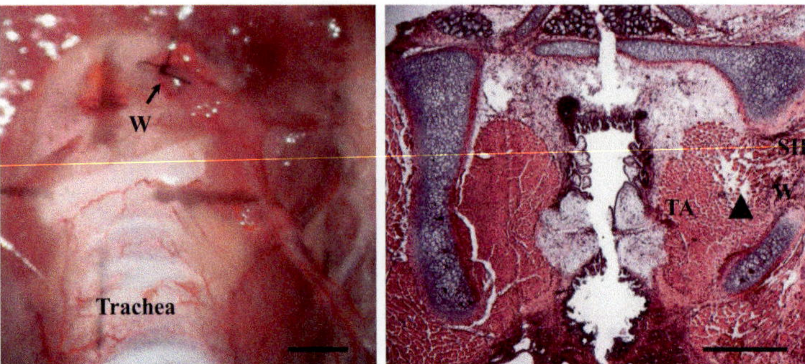

Fig. 3.15 Nerve–muscle pedicle flap implantation. *Left*: The nerve–muscle pedicle flap is sutured with 10-0 nylon to the exposed thyroarytenoid (*TA*) muscle through a window (*W*) created in the thyroid cartilage. The implanted flap passes through the window. Scale bar: 1 mm. *Right*: Representative histology of a coronal section of a rat taken 10 weeks after nerve–muscle pedicle (*NMP*) implantation. The *arrowhead* indicates the site of NMP transplantation. Scale bar: 1 mm. *W* window made in the thyroid cartilage, *SH* the sternohyoid muscle (Citation: Ref. [59])

allowed to recover in an approved animal care facility. After 2, 4, and 10 weeks (six animals per group), the rats were killed by intraperitoneal administration of an overdose of pentobarbital. The muscle areas and NMJ numbers were evaluated as described in Sect. 3.2.1.

To identify the MyHC isoforms present in the TA and SH muscles, immunohistochemistry was performed using two mouse monoclonal antibodies specific for MyHC type 2A (clone SC-71) and MyHC type 2B (clone BF-F3). The proportion of muscle fibers expressing MyHC type 2A and type 2B was quantified on photomicrographs of stained tissue sections (600 fibers were counted in each animal). To further evaluate the expression levels of MyHC of types 2A and 2B, reverse-transcriptase polymerase chain reaction (RT-PCR) was performed on samples obtained via laser capture microdissection (LCM). Nine female 8-week-old Wistar rats were used in this experiment, and the animals were divided into three groups: control, 10-week DNV, and 10-week NMP groups. Each larynx was isolated and cut with a cryostat to obtain frozen coronal sections 5 μm thick. Figure 3.16 shows representative microscopic features of the TA muscle before (B) and after (C) clipping of targeted samples via LCM [59].

3.3.1.1 Areas of Entire TA Muscle and Individual Muscle Fibers

In the DNV group, both the total area of the TA muscle and that of individual muscle fibers decreased gradually over time (Figs. 3.17 and 3.18). In contrast, in the NMP group, both indices significantly decreased at 2 weeks (compared to control, $P < 0.01$) and gradually recovered at 10 weeks (to 96.8 ± 6.2 % and 101.1 ± 18.5 % of control values, respectively). The latter values did not significantly differ from those of the controls (Figs. 3.17 and 3.18).

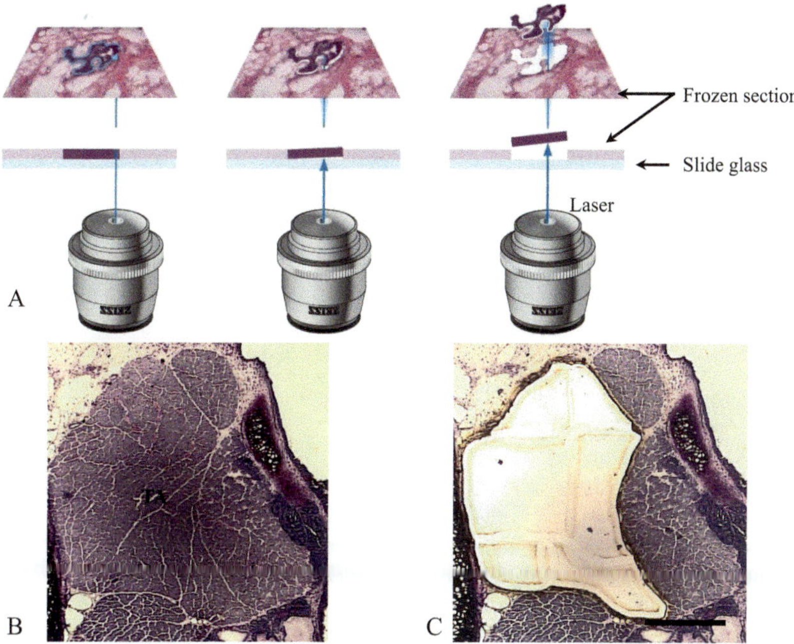

Fig. 3.16 Harvesting of targeted samples (the thyroarytenoid [*TA*] muscle stained with toluidine blue) using laser capture microdissection (*LCM*) prior to reverse-transcriptase polymerase chain reaction analysis of myosin heavy chain expression levels. (**A**) Schematic illustration of how to harvest targeted samples (TA muscle) from microscopic tissue slice by LCM method. Left; Start to isolate the border of the TA muscle under microscopic control, center; Isolate the targeted tissue, and right; harvest the targeted tissue for further analysis Microscopic findings before (**B**) and after (**C**) clipping of samples. Scale bar: 1 mm (Citation: Ref. [59])

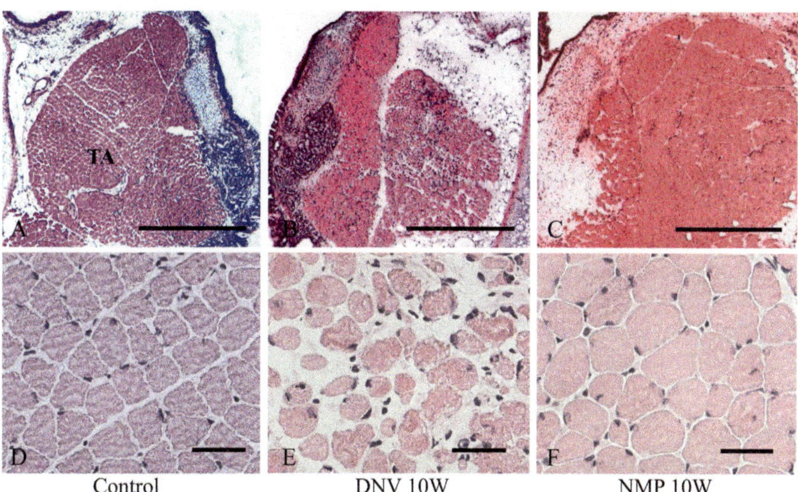

Fig. 3.17 Microscopic findings on the thyroarytenoid (*TA*) muscle. **A** and **D**, control groups. **B** and **E**, DNV groups analyzed 10 weeks after transection of the left recurrent laryngeal nerve (*RLN*). **C** and **F**, NMP groups analyzed 10 weeks after transection of the left RLN with implantation of an NMP. Scale bars: **A**, **B**, and **C** 1 mm; **D**, **E**, and **F** 50 μm (Citation: Ref. [59])

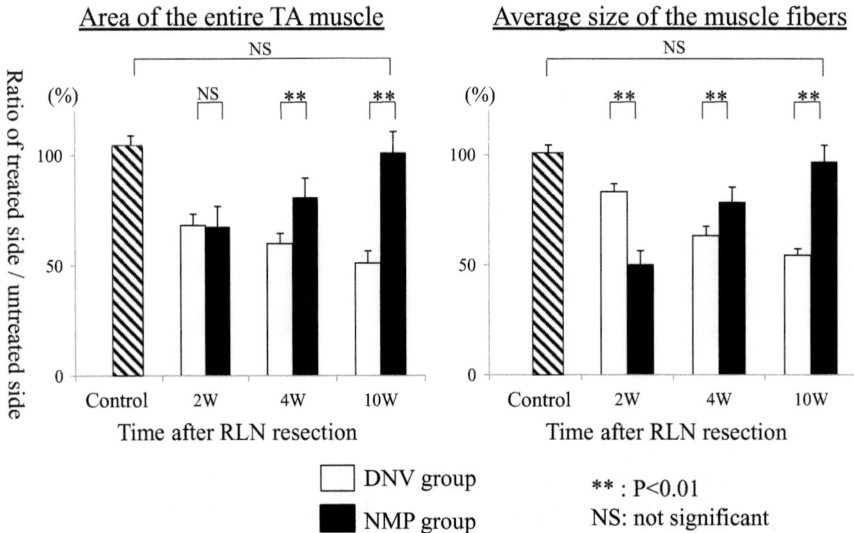

Fig. 3.18 Temporal changes in the treated/untreated (*T/U*) ratios of the areas of the entire TA muscle (*left*) and of individual muscle fibers (*right*) in the DNV (*white bars*) and NMP (*black bars*) groups after transection of the left recurrent laryngeal nerve (*RLN*). All data are presented as means ± SDs (Citation: Ref. [59])

3.3.1.2   The Neuromuscular Junction

In the DNV group, all nerve terminals disappeared by 2 weeks post-denervation. In contrast, in the NMP group, the proportion of nerve terminals compared to the number of AchRs at 2 weeks was 12.6 ± 31.2 % (P < 0.01 vs. control), and this proportion gradually increased. At 10 weeks, the NMP group ratio attained 79.8 ± 11.8 % (P < 0.05 vs. control) (Figs. 3.19 and 3.20).

3.3.1.3   The Myosin Heavy Chain Isoform

In the SH muscle, a portion of which had been used to construct the NMP flap, MyHC of types 2A and 2B constituted 28.5 ± 4.2 % and 51.1 ± 3.8 % of all evaluated fibers, respectively (Fig. 3.21). MyHC type 2B fibers were detected in the TA muscle of the control group, but MyHC type 2A fibers were not (Fig. 3.22 A, E). In the DNV group, as in the controls, only MyHC type 2B fibers were evident between 4 and 10 weeks, and the number of such fibers gradually decreased to 88.4 ± 5.7 % of all fibers counted at 10 weeks (P < 0.05 vs. control). In the NMP group, in contrast to the control and DNV groups, MyHC type 2A fibers appeared at 4 weeks (1.9 ± 0.4 %) and significantly increased in number at 10 weeks to constitute 14.3 ± 0.8 % of all fibers counted (P < 0.05 vs. the 4-week level). Between 4 and 10 weeks, MyHC type 2B fibers gradually decreased in number and at 10 weeks

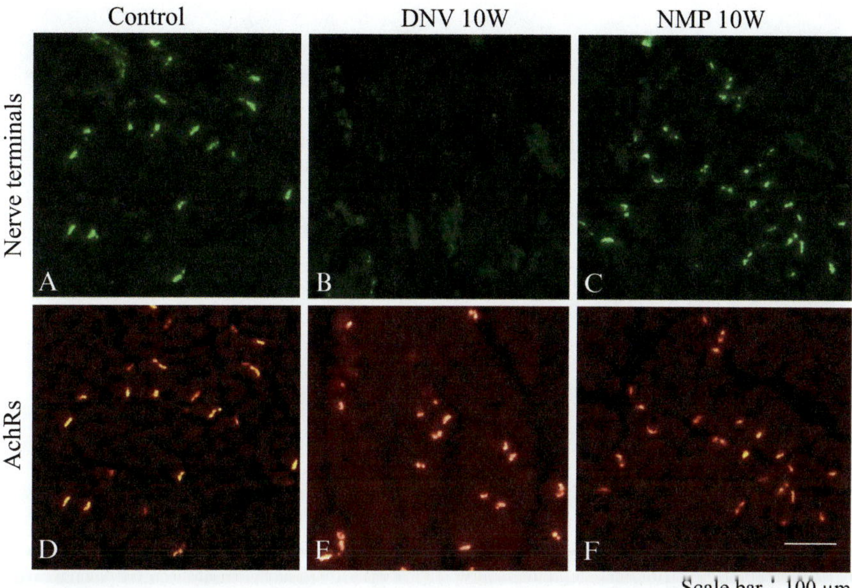

Fig. 3.19 Representative microscopic images of neuromuscular junctions (*NMJs*) in the rat thyroarytenoid (*TA*) muscle. **A** and **D**, control; **B** and **E**, DNV group analyzed 10 weeks after transection of the recurrent laryngeal nerve (*RLN*), **C** and **F**, NMP group analyzed 10 weeks after an NMP flap was implanted following RLN transection. In the DNV animals, although acetylcholine receptors (*AchRs*) persisted (**E**), all nerve terminals disappeared (**B**). In contrast, in NMP animals, the locations of nerve terminals and AchRs matched (**C, F**), as was also true of control animals (Citation: Ref. [59])

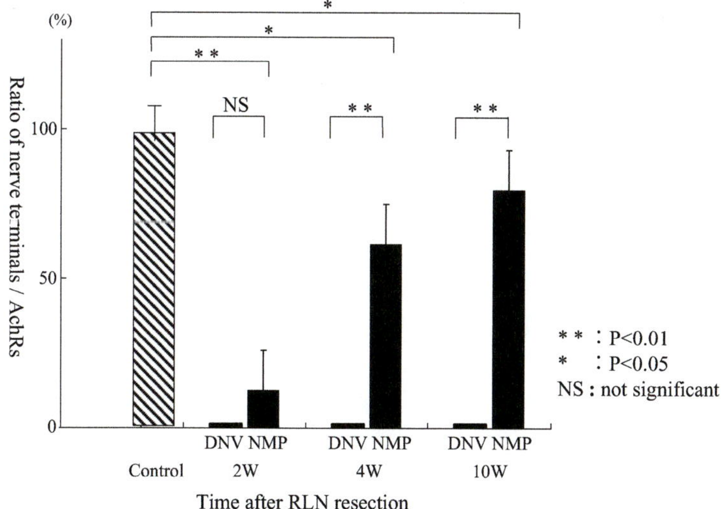

Fig. 3.20 Temporal changes in the ratios of the numbers of nerve terminals compared to those of acetylcholine receptors (*AchRs*) in the thyroarytenoid muscle in the DNV (*white bars*) and NMP (*black bars*) groups. All data are presented as means ± SDs (Citation: Ref. [59])

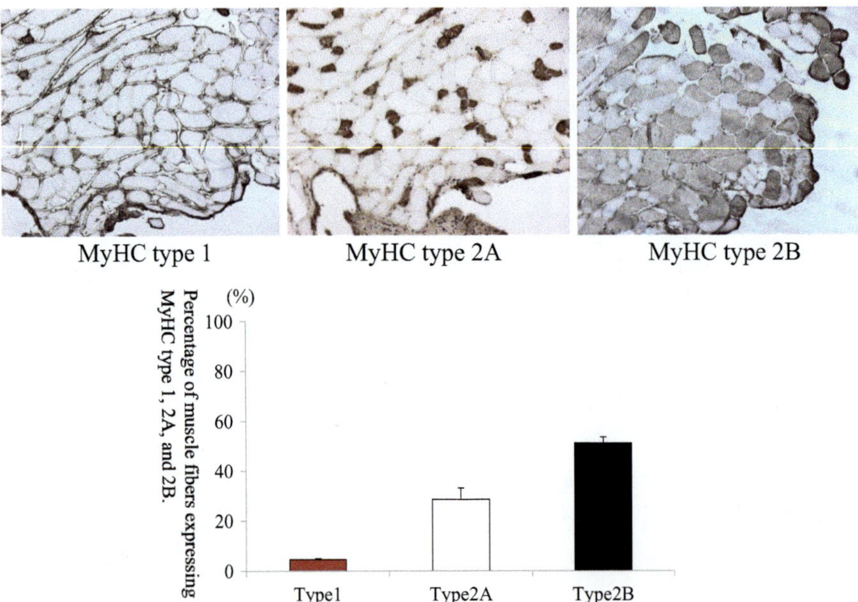

Fig. 3.21 Myosin heavy chain (*MyHC*) expression levels, determined immunohistochemically, in the rat sternohyoid muscle. All data are presented as means ± SDs

reached 81.3 ± 8.2 % of the total (P < 0.05 vs. control), similar to the DNV group (Figs. 3.22, 3.23, and 3.24). RT-PCR data on the TA muscle confirmed that the MyHC type 2A isoform was only present in the NMP group, whereas the MyHC type 2B isoform was present in all of the control, DNV, and NMP groups (Fig. 3.25).

The partial replacement of the faster MyHC type 2B by the slower type 2A (the "fast-to-slow twitch") has been demonstrated in experimental models exploring enhanced neuromuscular activity [60] and changes in NMJs that affect muscle fiber phenotype [61]. Therefore, the observed fiber transformation in the NMP group of the present study may reflect successful reinnervation via a novel neural input from the ACN branch.

3.3.2 Delayed Implantation

As described in Sect. 3.3.1, NMP flap implantation performed immediately after denervation effectively enhanced recovery of the denervated rat TA muscle, protecting the muscle from atrophic changes. However, long-term observations until 58 weeks after denervation showed that the number of AchRs decreased gradually, commencing 10 weeks after denervation. Thus, the ability of a denervated TA muscle to accommodate regenerating nerve axons may decline over time, and a reinnervated muscle may not regain adequate functionality after prolonged denervation. In clinical situations, we often treat patients who have suffered from UVFP for months

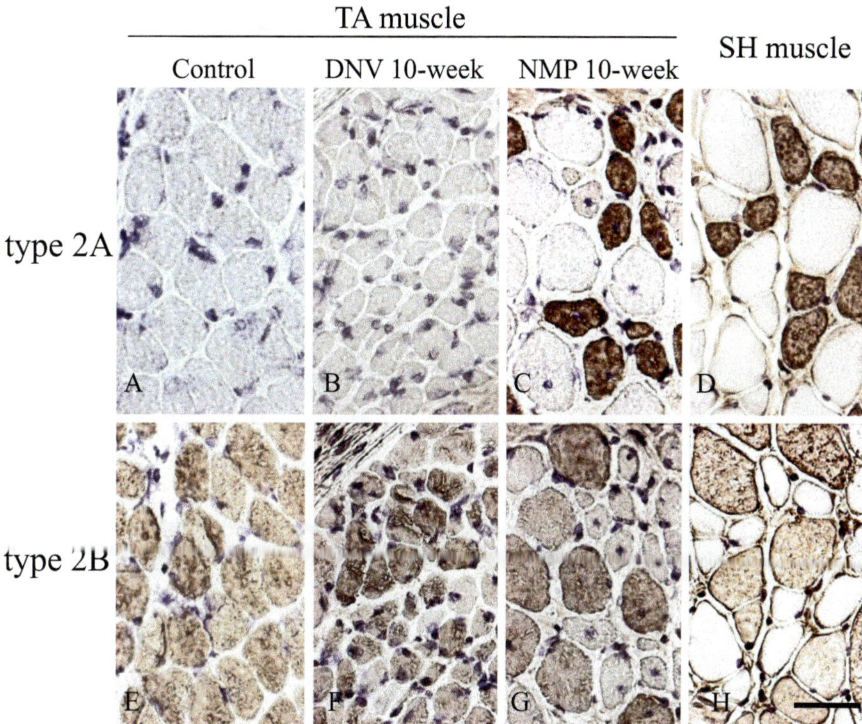

Fig. 3.22 Myosin heavy chain (*MyHC*) expression levels, determined immunohistochemically in the thyroarytenoid (*TA*) muscles of three experimental groups (**A**, **E**, control group; **B**, **F**, DNV 10-week group; **C**, **G**, NMP 10-week group) and in the sternohyoid (*SH*) muscle (**D**, **H**), using an anti-MyHC type 2A antibody (**A**, **B**, **C**, and **D**) and an anti-MyHC type 2B antibody (**E**, **F**, **G**, and **H**). Scale bar: 50 μm (Citation: Ref. [59])

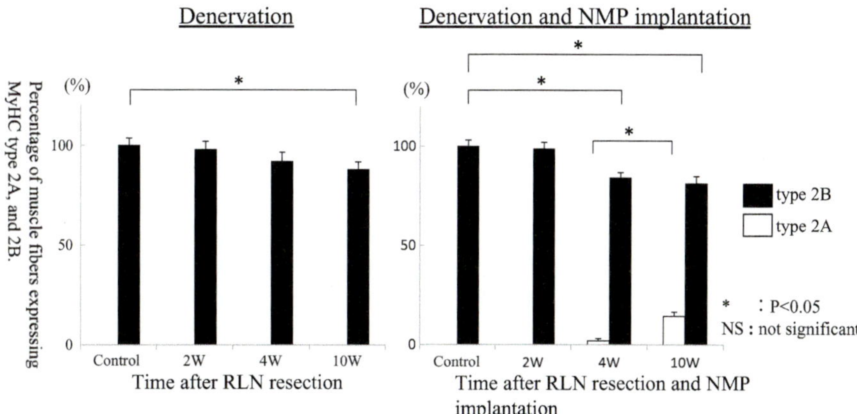

Fig. 3.23 Temporal changes in myosin heavy chain (*MyHC*) expression levels in thyroarytenoid (*TA*) muscle fibers after recurrent laryngeal nerve (*RLN*) transection alone (*left*) and RLN transection with nerve–muscle pedicle (*NMP*) implantation (*right*). All data are presented as means ± SDs (Citation: Ref. [59])

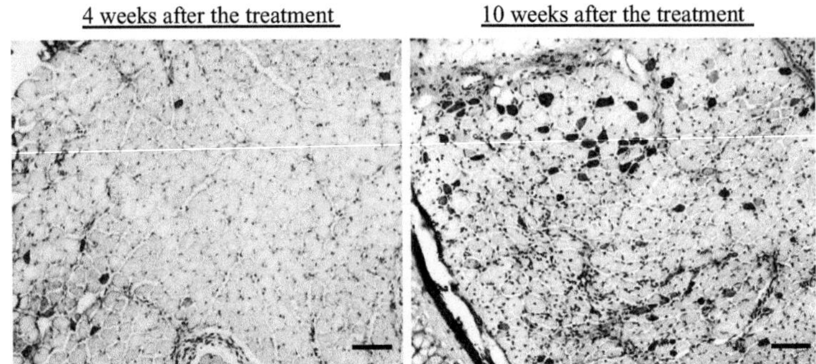

Fig. 3.24 The increase in the level of myosin heavy chain (*MyHC*) type 2A expression in thyroarytenoid (*TA*) muscle fibers 10 weeks after recurrent laryngeal nerve (*RLN*) resection and nerve–muscle pedicle (*NMP*) flap implantation, compared to the level 4 weeks after such treatment. Scale bar: 100 μm (Citation: Ref. [59])

Fig. 3.25 Representative reverse-transcriptase polymerase chain reaction data on the expression levels of three types of myosin heavy chain (2A, 2B, 2X) and β-actin in the thyroarytenoid muscles of the control, DNV, and NMP groups (Citation: Ref. [59])

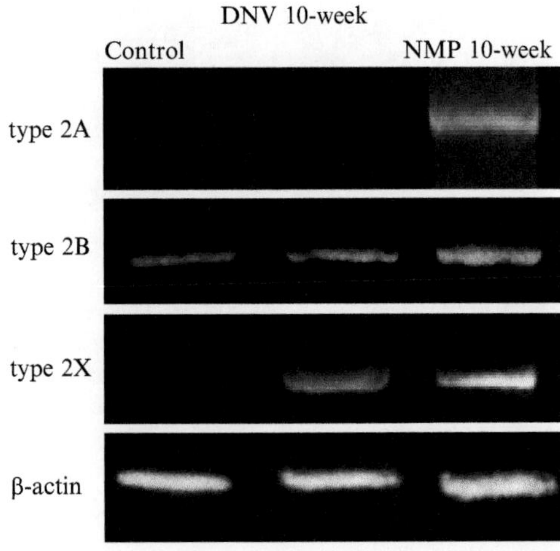

or years. In addition, when the extent of injury to the RLN is unknown, we usually manage patients conservatively, monitoring them closely for about 6 months. Only after such a period has elapsed can we establish a rational treatment plan and decide whether to proceed with surgical intervention. It remains to be clarified whether NMP flap implantation after long-term denervation effectively reinnervates the TA muscle. In this section, the effects of NMP treatment on long-term denervated rat TA muscle will be quantitatively described in histological and physiological terms.

The methods used for RLN resection and NMP implantation were described above (Sect. 3.3.1). We formed five NMP subgroups, animals that were implanted immediately after RLN resection and 8, 16, 32, and 48 weeks thereafter; each group had 14 animals. Ten weeks after NMP implantation, EMG was performed on seven animals of each subgroup to explore reinnervation via the ACN, and the other seven rats were euthanized prior to histological evaluation of TA muscle areas and NMJ numbers. Animals in the five DNV subgroups were euthanized at 10, 18, 26, 42, and

58 weeks after RLN resection, for histological evaluation. Next, we compared experimental data between the NMP and DNV subgroups paired in the sense that the elapsed time after RLN transection was the same. For example, 10 weeks after NMP implantation, the NMP subgroup implanted 48 weeks after denervation (termed 48 + 10) was matched with the DNV subgroup 58 weeks after denervation [62].

3.3.2.1   Areas of the Entire TA Muscle and Individual Muscle Fibers

Figure 3.26 shows representative microscopic findings on the TA muscle of the control, DNV 58, and NMP 48 + 10 groups. Figure 3.27 shows temporal changes in the T/U ratios of entire muscle areas and those of individual muscle fibers. In the DNV group, the entire TA muscle area of the treated side was less than that of the untreated side. The areas of individual muscle fibers of the treated side were also less than those of the untreated side. In contrast, the areas of individual muscle fibers in the NMP group were widely distributed, and almost half were the same as those of the untreated side. In addition, some muscle fibers had nuclei in the center of the cytoplasm (central nuclei muscle fibers). The T/U ratios for the entire TA muscle area in four of the five NMP subgroups were significantly greater than those of the corresponding DNV subgroups (P<0.01 or P<0.05). In all of the NMP subgroups, the T/U ratios of individual muscle fiber areas were significantly greater

Control   DNV 58 weeks   NMP 48+10 weeks

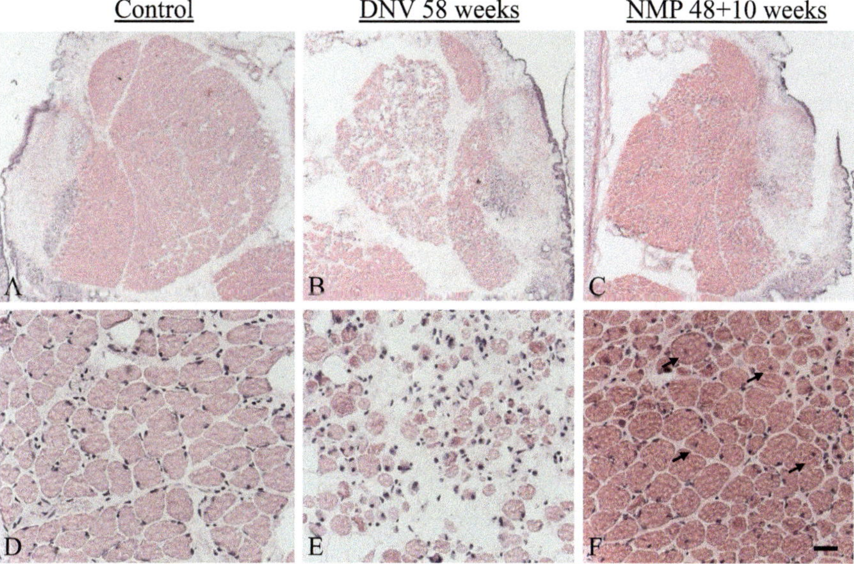

Fig. 3.26 Representative microscopic images of the thyroarytenoid muscle. **A** and **D**, control; **B** and **E**, 58 weeks after resection of the recurrent laryngeal nerve (*RLN*); **C** and **F**, 10 weeks after NMP implantation at a time 48 weeks after resection of the RLN. *Arrows* indicate nuclei located in the center of the cytoplasm, thus not close to the cell membrane. Scale bars: **A**, **B**, and **C** 200 μm; **D**, **E**, and **F** 20 μm (Citation: Ref. [62])

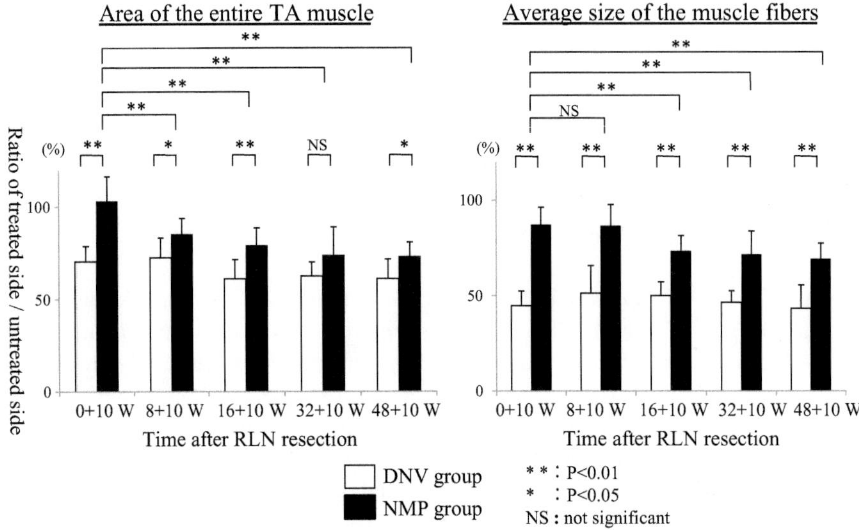

Fig. 3.27 Temporal changes in the treated/untreated (*T/U*) ratios of the areas of the entire TA muscle (*left*) and those of individual muscle fibers (*right*) in DNV (*white bars*) and NMP (*black bars*) groups after transection of the recurrent laryngeal nerve (*RLN*). All data are presented as means ± SDs (Citation: Ref. [62])

than those of the DNV subgroups (P < 0.01). Of the five NMP subgroups, the T/U ratio of the entire muscle area of the 0 + 10 subgroup was significantly greater than those of the other four subgroups (P < 0.01). The T/U ratio of individual muscle fiber area was significantly greater in the 0 + 10 subgroup than in the subgroups undergoing NMP implantation more than 16 weeks after RLN transection (P < 0.01).

3.3.2.2   Central-Nuclei Muscle Fibers

In all NMP subgroups, the incidence of central-nuclei muscle fibers was significantly greater on the treated than the untreated side, except in the 0 + 10 subgroup (Fig. 3.28). When the indices of treated sides were compared, those of the 0 + 10 and 8 + 10 subgroups were significantly lower than those of the other three subgroups, and the ratio of the 0 + 10 subgroup was significantly lower than that of the 8 + 10 subgroup.

3.3.2.3   The Neuromuscular Junction

Although AchRs persisted in long-term denervated TA muscle, the AchRs were shrunken and distorted (Fig. 3.29). The ratios of nerve terminal to AchR numbers in the NMP subgroups were significantly higher than those of the corresponding DNV subgroups up to 32 weeks after denervation (Fig. 3.30). In the 48 + 10 subgroups, the ratio

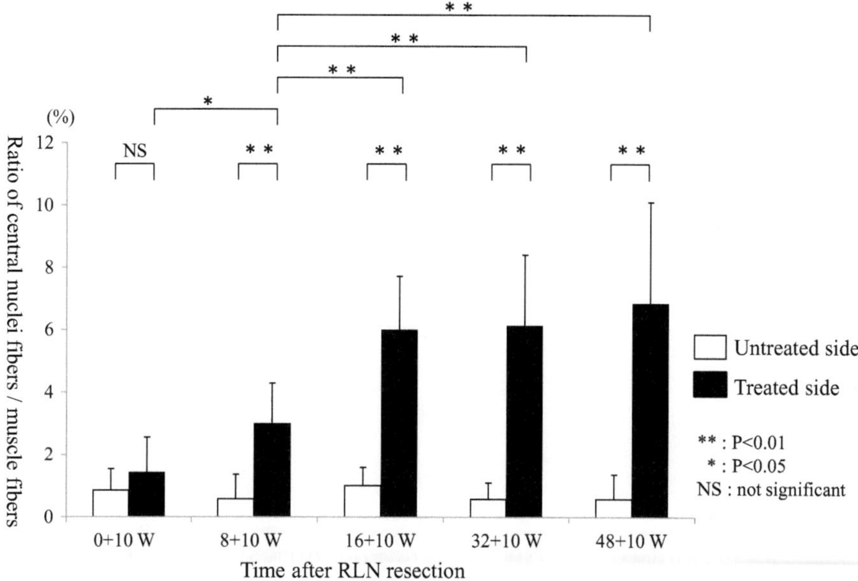

Fig. 3.28 Temporal changes in the ratios of muscle fibers (100 were evaluated) containing nuclei in the center of the cytoplasm in the untreated (*U*) (*white bars*) and treated (*T*) (*black bars*) thyroarytenoid muscles of the NMP subgroups. All data are presented as means ± SDs (Citation: Ref. [62])

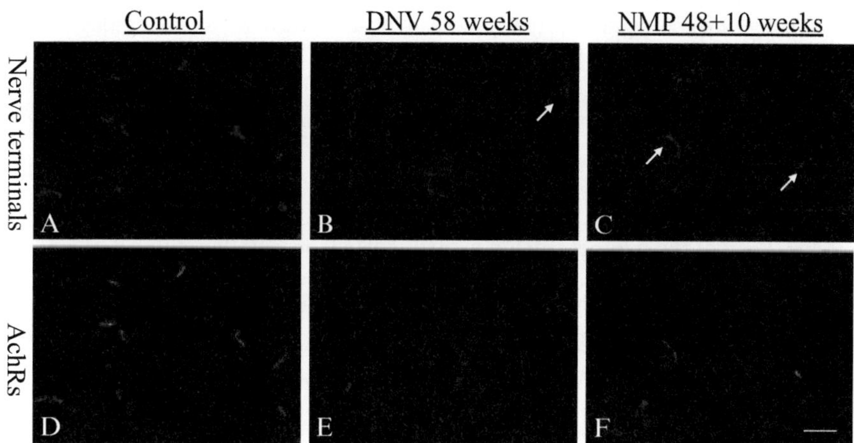

Fig. 3.29 Representative microscopic images of neuromuscular junctions in the thyroarytenoid muscle. **A** and **D**, control; **B** and **E**, the DNV 58-week subgroup; **C** and **F**, the NMP 48 + 10 week subgroup. *Arrows* indicate nerve terminals, the locations of which correspond to the locations of acetylcholine receptors (*AchRs*). Scale bar: 20 µm (Citation: Ref. [62])

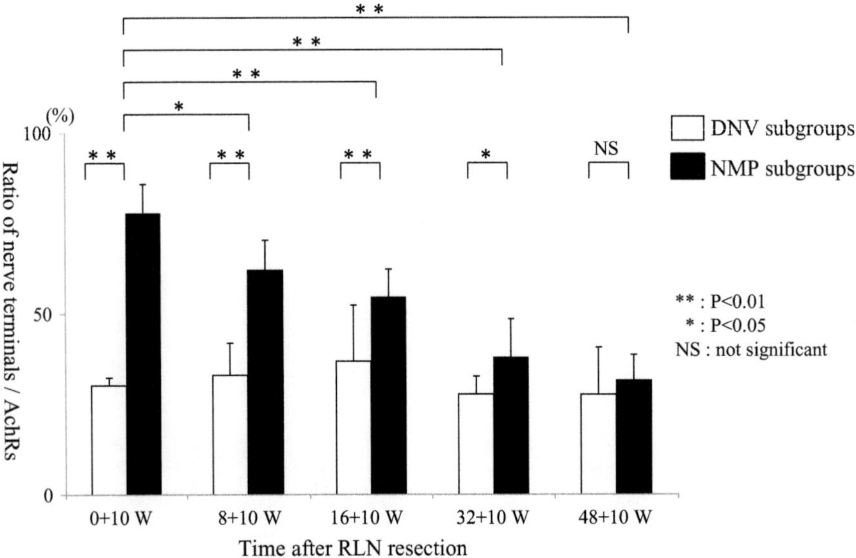

Fig. 3.30 Temporal changes in the ratios of the numbers of nerve terminals to those of acetylcholine receptors (*AchRs*) in the thyroarytenoid muscle of the DNV (*white bars*) and NMP (*black bars*) subgroups. All data are presented as means ± SDs (Citation: Ref. [62])

in the NMP subgroup was somewhat higher than that of the DNV subgroup, although statistical significance was not attained. Among the NMP subgroups, the ratio of the 0 + 10 subgroup was significantly higher than those of the other four subgroups.

3.3.2.4 Evoked Electromyographic Data

Evoked TA muscle action potentials were evident in all NMP-treated animals. No muscle activity was elicited after the transferred ACN was cut (Fig. 3.31). When the proximal end of the transected RLN was stimulated, no muscle activity was evident, indicating that no EMG-detectable reinnervation occurred via the transected RLN. The T/U ratio of the evoked action potential decreased as the time from RLN transection to NMP implantation increased (Fig. 3.32). The 0 + 10 subgroup had a significantly greater evoked action potential T/U ratio than the 16 + 10 or 48 + 10 subgroups.

3.3.2.5 The Denervation Period Affects Reinnervation
of the TA Muscle Using the NMP Method

The TA muscle becomes atrophic after denervation, but as described in Sect. 3.3.1, the muscle can recover if NMP flap implantation is performed immediately after resection of the RLN. Section 3.3.2 also showed that the NMP method could be

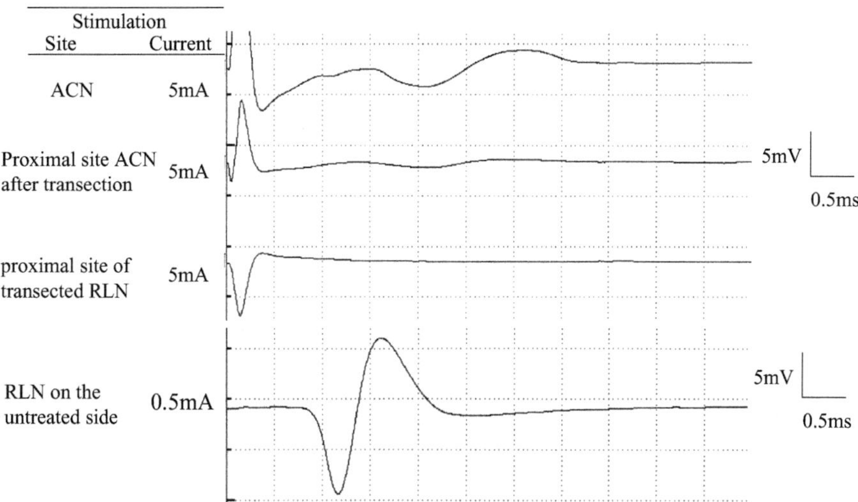

Fig. 3.31 Representative evoked electromyographic potentials of the left thyroarytenoid muscle in the NMP 8 + 10 subgroup and controls (*right side*). The *upper row* is a waveform obtained upon stimulation of the transferred ansa cervicalis nerve (*ACN*). The *second row* is a waveform obtained upon stimulation of the central site after transection of the ACN. The *third row* is a waveform obtained upon stimulation of the proximal site of the transected left RLN. The *bottom row* is a waveform obtained upon stimulation of the right RLN (Citation: Ref. [62])

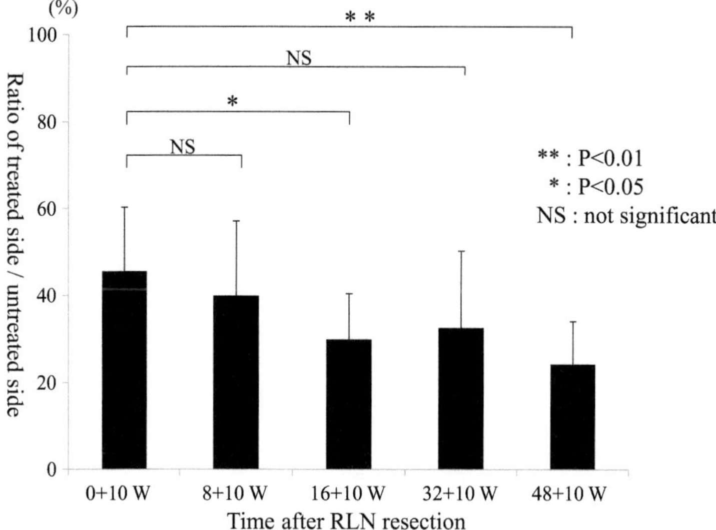

Fig. 3.32 Temporal changes in the treated/untreated (*T/U*) ratios of the action potentials of the thyroarytenoid muscles in the NMP subgroups. All data are presented as means ± SDs (Citation: Ref. [62])

effectively used to assist recovery of a denervated TA muscle from atrophic changes until at least 48 weeks after denervation. Functional restoration of the TA muscle after long-term denervation was also shown by the presence of evoked action potentials upon stimulation of the transferred ACN. These experiments were performed in a rat model. Considering the life span of the rat (2.5–3 years), the 48-week duration of denervation in the rat may correspond to more than 10 years of human life. Thus, reinnervation of a denervated TA muscle may be possible even after years of VFP.

In the rat model, the outcome afforded by the NMP method applied to a denervated TA muscle became poorer as the time from denervation to NMP flap application increased. Nguyen et al. [63] found that during reinnervation, axons extended to the residual AchRs. Thus, the ability of a denervated TA muscle to receive regenerating axons may gradually decline over time after denervation. Structural changes in skeletal muscle AchRs after denervation (Fig. 3.29) may render the muscle inadequately functional, even if regenerating fibers in fact reach the muscle [45]. However, AchR size was not reduced in the NMP group (Figs. 3.29 and 3.35). Sprouting nerve terminals can form new NMJs at or near the locations of original NMJs when the latter disappear after prolonged denervation [64]. Thus, when regenerating nerve fibers reach the denervated muscle, new NMJs may form.

Because newly fused satellite cell nuclei are initially centrally located in regenerated myofibrils, migrating later to more peripheral locations [65], the presence of central-nuclei muscle fibers (Figs. 3.26 and 3.28) may indicate that the fibers of the denervated TA muscle were not yet fully mature, and thus, the effectiveness of the NMP method may gradually increase over a time period longer than 10 weeks after NMP implantation. Consequently, in instances of prolonged denervation, the effects of the NMP method may be greater if the evaluation period after NMP flap implantation is longer than 10 weeks.

3.3.3   NMP Flap Implantation into the TA Muscle of the Aged Rat

As populations age worldwide, the number of elderly patients suffering from paralytic dysphonia is expected to increase rapidly. Some studies have explored age-associated negative changes in size, conformation, and function of the laryngeal muscles [67–71]. Such changes may negatively affect reinnervation after NMP flap implantation in older patients.

In this section, the outcomes of NMP flap placement into the denervated TA muscle of aged rats will be described. Denervation and NMP models for both 20-month-old (aged) and 8-week-old (young) rats used the same method as described in the previous section. Ten weeks after treatment, evoked EMG was performed on each NMP subgroup ($n = 5$), and the remaining rats ($n = 5$ in each subgroup) were euthanized for histological evaluation of muscle regions and the NMJs of the TA muscle. The aged rats were also evaluated 20 weeks after treatment (referred to as the aged NMP20 group) [66].

3.3.3.1   Areas of the Entire Muscle and Single Muscle Fibers

Figures 3.33 and 3.34 show the areas of the entire TA muscle and individual muscle fibers thereof. The T/U ratios of these areas in the aged NMP groups were significantly greater than those of the aged DNV groups ($P<0.01$). When the aged NMP group was compared to the young NMP group, the T/U ratio of the entire muscle area in the former group was significantly lower than that of the latter group ($P<0.05$), whereas no significant difference was evident between the aged NMP20 group and the young NMP10 group. The T/U ratios of individual muscle fiber areas in aged NMP groups were almost the same as those of the young NMP group.

3.3.3.2   The Neuromuscular Junction

Figures 3.35, 3.36, and 3.37 show data on nerve terminals and AchRs. The T/U ratios of nerve terminal numbers in the aged NMP groups were significantly higher than those of the aged DNV groups ($P<0.01$). The T/U ratios of AchR numbers were significantly greater in the aged NMP20 group than in the aged DNV20 group ($P<0.05$) (Fig. 3.36). The nerve terminal/AchR ratios were significantly higher in the aged NMP groups than in the aged DNV groups ($P<0.01$). When the aged NMP groups and the young NMP groups were compared, no significant differences were observed in the T/U ratios of nerve terminal or AchR numbers, or nerve terminal/AchR ratios.

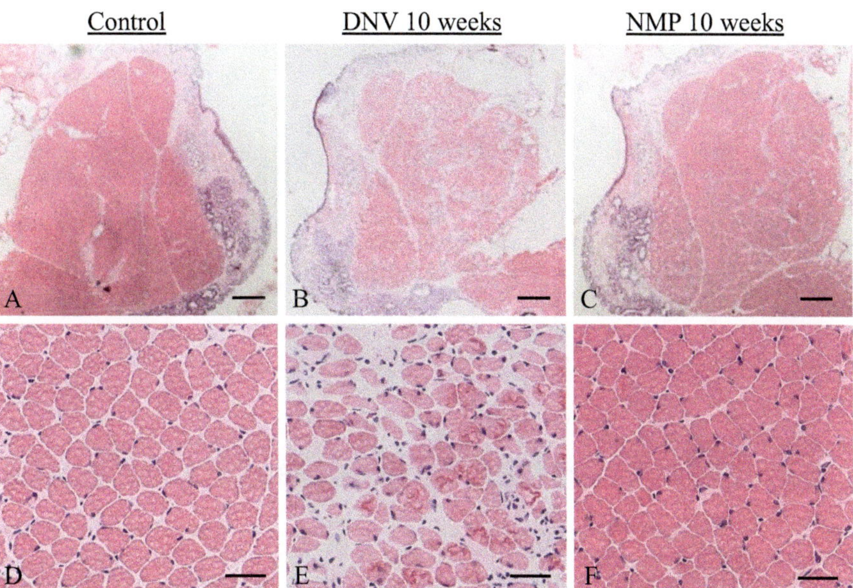

Fig. 3.33 Representative microscopic images of the thyroarytenoid muscle of aged rats. **A** and **D**, control; **B** and **E**, 10 weeks after resection of the recurrent laryngeal nerve (DNV); **C** and **F**, 10 weeks after NMP implantation (NMP). Scale bars: **A**, **B**, and **C** 200 µm; **D**, **E**, and **F** 20 µm

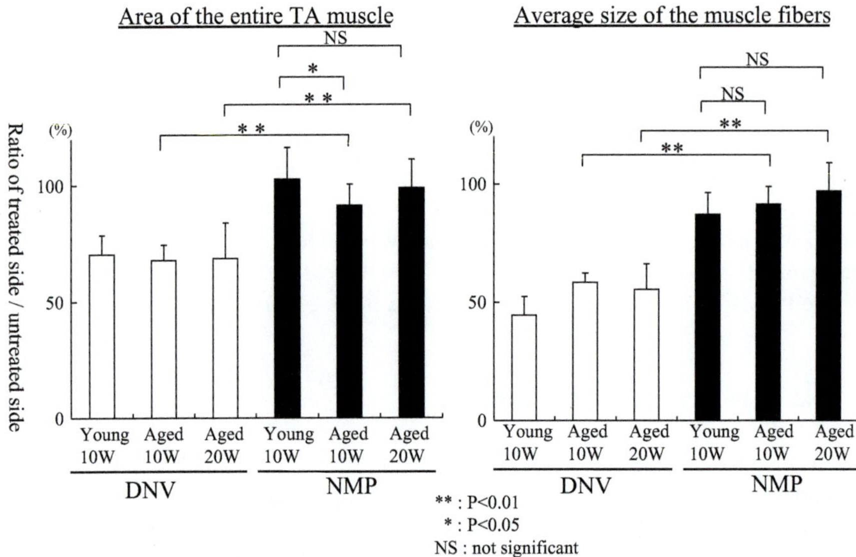

Fig. 3.34 Temporal changes in the treated/untreated (*T/U*) ratios of the areas of the entire TA muscle (*left*) and of individual muscle fibers (*right*) in DNV (*white bars*) and NMP (*black bars*) groups of both young and old rats. All data are presented as means ± SDs (Citation: Ref. [66])

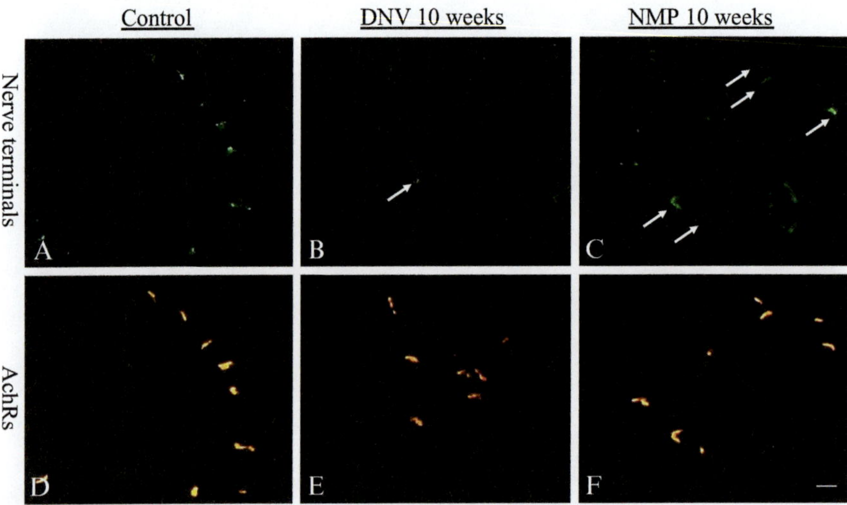

Fig. 3.35 Representative microscopic images of neuromuscular junctions in the thyroarytenoid muscle of aged rats. **A** and **D**, controls; **B** and **E**, DNV 10-week subgroup; **C** and **FD**, NMP 10-week subgroup. *Arrows* indicate nerve terminals, the locations of which correspond to those of acetylcholine receptors (*AchRs*). Scale bar: 20 μm

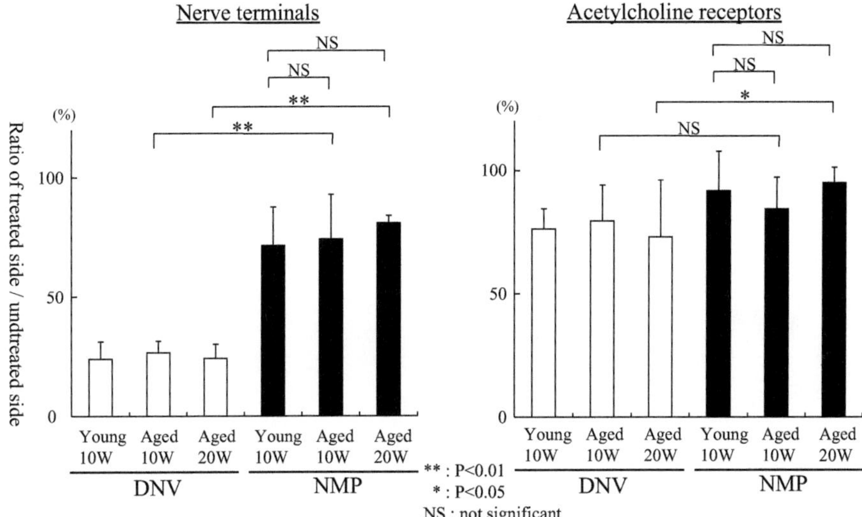

Fig. 3.36 Temporal changes in the treated/untreated ratios of the numbers of nerve terminals (*left*) and acetylcholine receptors (*right*) in DNV (*white bars*) and NMP (*black bars*) groups of both young and old rats. All data are presented as means ± SDs (Citation: Ref. [66])

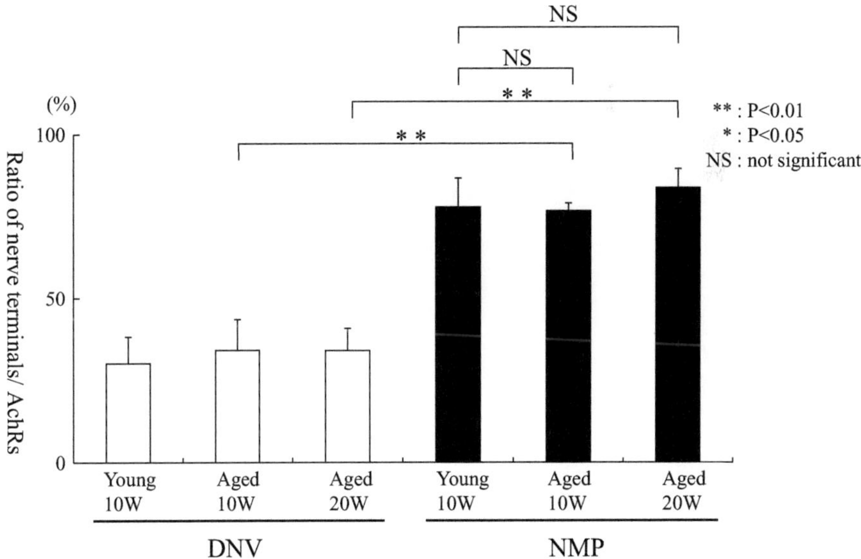

Fig. 3.37 Temporal changes in the ratios of the number of nerve terminals to those of acetylcholine receptors (*AchRs*) in the thyroarytenoid muscles of the DNV (*white bars*) and NMP (*black bars*) subgroups of both young and old rats. All data are presented as means ± SDs (Citation: Ref. [66])

3.3.3.3 Evoked Electromyography

When the transferred ACN was stimulated, evoked action potentials of the TA muscle were seen in all NMP animals (Fig. 3.38). No muscle activity was elicited after the transferred ACN was cut. When the proximal end of the transected RLN was stimulated, no muscle activity was evident, indicating that no EMG-detectable reinnervation occurred via the transected RLN. The T/U ratios of the action potentials of the aged NMP groups did not differ significantly from those of the young NMP group (Fig. 3.39).

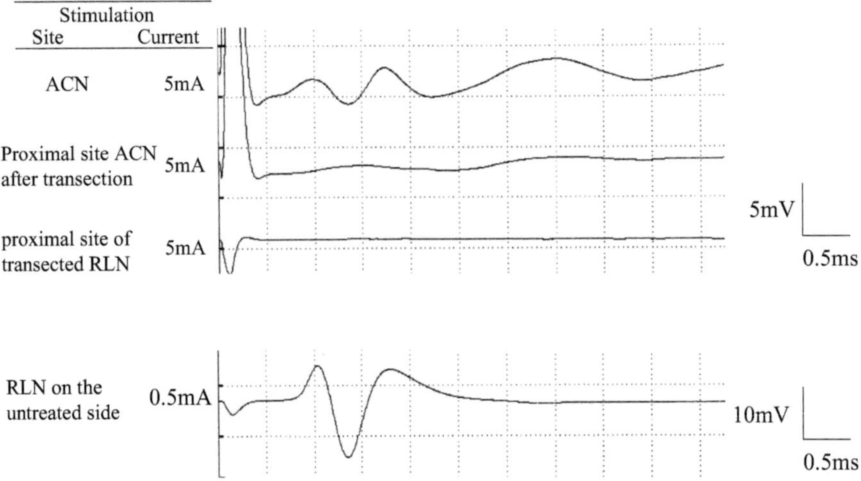

Fig. 3.38 Representative evoked electromyographic potentials of the thyroarytenoid muscle in the aged NMP 10 model. The *upper row* is a waveform obtained upon stimulation of the transferred ansa cervicalis nerve (*ACN*). The *second row* is a waveform obtained upon stimulation of the proximal site of the ACN after transection. The *third row* is a waveform obtained upon stimulation of the proximal site of the transected left recurrent laryngeal nerve (*RLN*). The *bottom row* is a waveform obtained upon stimulation of the right RLN

Fig. 3.39 Temporal changes in the treated/untreated (*T/U*) ratio of the action potential of the thyroarytenoid muscle in the aged NMP model. All data are presented as means ± SDs (Citation: Ref. [66])

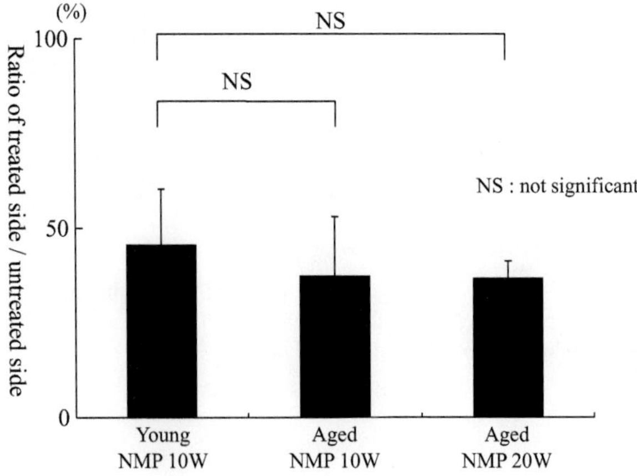

In summary, when young and aged NMP groups were compared, no significant difference was observed either histologically or physiologically, except that the entire TA muscle area differed between the young and aged NMP10 groups. This difference is explained by development of connective tissue among muscle fibers, because the individual muscle fiber area did not differ between the young and aged NMP10 groups. These data suggest that the NMP method is equally effective for young and aged animals, rendering the NMP method effective when used to remedy atrophic changes in the denervated TA muscle of aged rats. Thus, the NMP method may be useful in treating elderly patients suffering from paralytic dysphonia.

3.3.4   NMP Flap Implantation into the TA Muscle in the Presence of Partial Innervation

As previously reported, functionally active muscle fibers may not accept further innervation [72]. However, many RLN injuries suffered by UVFP patients cause only partial denervation, and reinnervation is associated with impairment of vocal fold motion to various extents, accompanied by weakness, synkinesis, and partial atrophy [74]. Thus, any effect of the NMP procedure on a TA muscle that is partially innervated is questionable. In this section, supply of a foreign nerve (the ACN) via performance of an NMP procedure on a partially innervated TA will be examined.

3.3.4.1   Animal Model

Eight-week female Wistar rats were used. In addition to a DNV group ($n=6$), another group was composed of animals in which, immediately after RLN transection, both nerve stumps were placed in a silicone tube (ST), held 1 mm apart, and fixed with 9-0 nylon sutures (24 animals). Of these, 12 animals underwent the NMP procedure 5 weeks after anastomosis (the NMP group). The other 12 animals underwent anastomosis alone (the ST group). Figure 3.40 shows the procedures performed on the ST and NMP groups. Each group was divided into two subgroups of six animals, of which one underwent histological analysis and the other measurement of evoked EMG potentials. Fifteen weeks after RLN resection, no spontaneous vocal fold movement was evident on the treated side of any animal in the DNV, ST, or NMP groups. Subsequently, histological and electromyographic analyses were performed [43, 73].

3.3.4.2   Areas of the Entire TA Muscle and Individual Muscle Fibers

In the NMP group, the entire TA muscle area and the area of individual muscle fibers on the treated side were larger than those of the DNV and ST groups (Fig. 3.41). The T/U ratio of the entire TA muscle area in the NMP group was

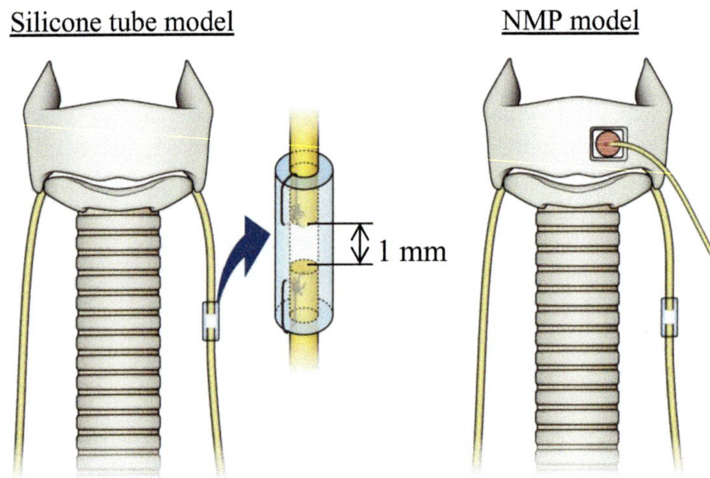

Fig. 3.40 The silicone tube (*ST*) model (*left*) and the nerve–muscle pedicle (*NMP*) model (*right*). The NMP procedure was performed 5 weeks after placement of nerve stumps in a silicone tube

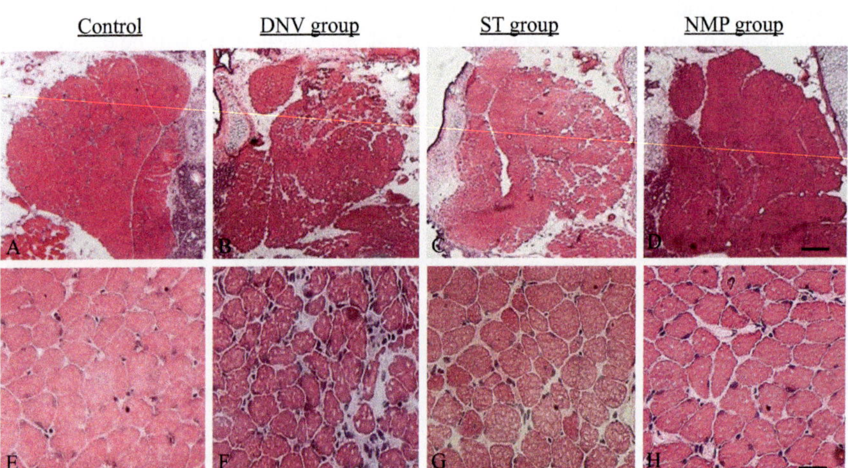

Fig. 3.41 Representative microscopic images of the thyroarytenoid muscle. **A** and **E**, control; **B** and **F**, 15 weeks after resection of the recurrent laryngeal nerve (DNV); **C** and **G**, the silicone tube (*ST*) group; **D** and **H**, the NMP implantation group. Scale bars: **A**, **B**, **C**, and **D** 200 μm; **E**, **F**, **G**, and **H** 20 μm (Modified from Ref. [43])

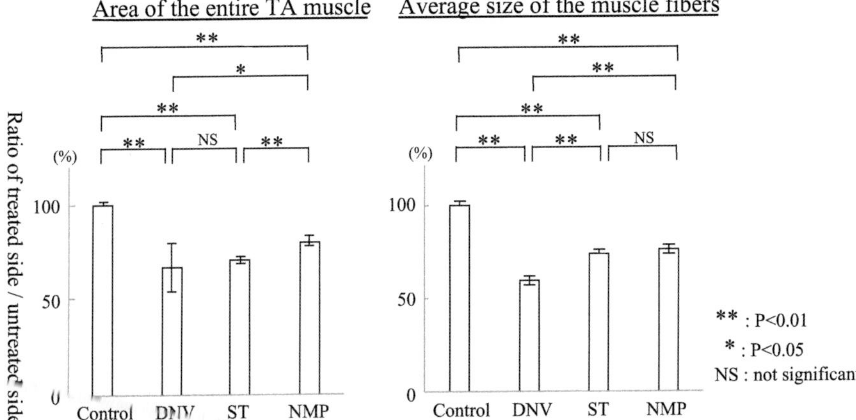

Fig. 3.42 Comparison of the treated/untreated (*T/U*) ratios of the areas of the entire TA muscle (*left*) and of individual muscle fibers (*right*) in the control, denervation (*DNV*), silicone tube (*ST*), and NMP groups. All data are presented as means ± SDs (Citation: Ref. [43])

significantly greater than that of the ST group (P<0.01) (Fig. 3.42; left). Although the difference did not attain statistical significance, the T/U ratio of the area of individual muscle fibers was slightly larger in the NMP group than in the ST group (P=0.051) (Fig. 3.42; right).

3.3.4.3 The Neuromuscular Junction

Figures 3.43, 3.44, and 3.45 show data on nerve terminals and AchRs, which were noted in all groups. The T/U ratios of the numbers of nerve terminals and AchRs, and the ratio of nerve terminal to AchR numbers in the NMP group, were significantly greater than those for the DNV and ST groups (P<0.01).

3.3.4.4 Evoked Electromyography

Figure 3.46 shows representative evoked EMG waveforms recorded from the TA muscle of the ST and NMP groups. Stimulation of the RLN at point (1) on the treated side evoked an EMG response, and after transection of the distal point at a, such a response was not elicited by stimulation at point (1), suggesting that the TA muscle was partially innervated by the RLN in both the ST and NMP groups. In the NMP group, when the ACN was stimulated at point (3), evoked potentials were noted. However, no muscle activity was elicited when the ACN distally transected at point b was stimulated at the same point (3).

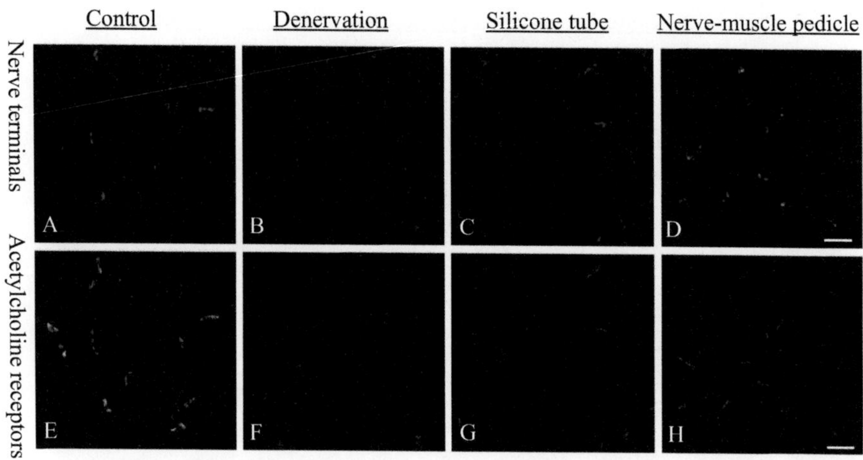

Fig. 3.43 Representative microscopic images of neuromuscular junctions in the thyroarytenoid muscle. **A** and **E**, controls; **B** and **F**, denervation group; **C** and **G**, silicone tube group; **D** and **H**, NMP group. Scale bar: 20 μm (Citation: Ref. [43])

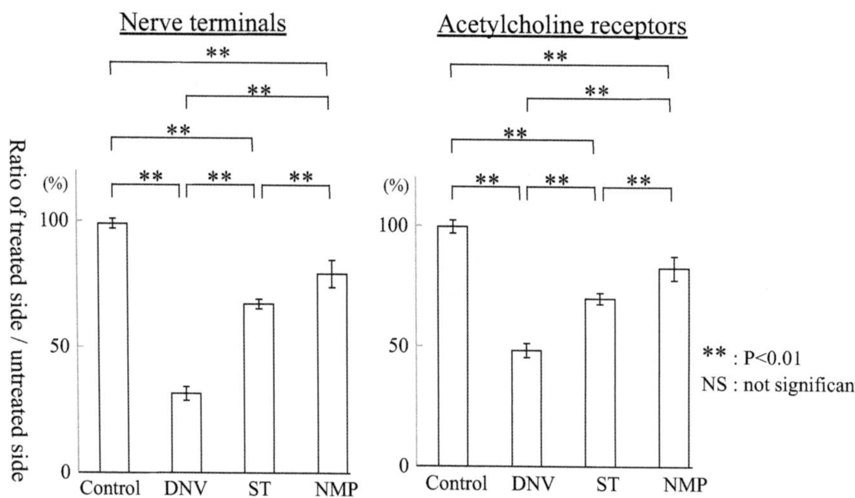

Fig. 3.44 Comparison of the treated/untreated ratios of the numbers of nerve terminals (*left*) and acetylcholine receptors (*right*) in the control, denervation (*DNV*), silicone tube (*ST*), and NMP groups. All data are presented as means ± SDs (Citation: Ref. [43])

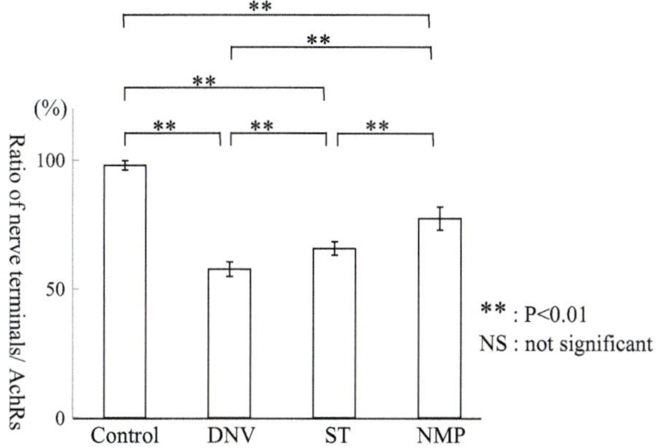

Fig. 3.45 Comparison of the ratios of the numbers of nerve terminals to those of acetylcholine receptors in the control, denervation (*DNV*), silicone tube (*ST*), and NMP groups. All data are presented as means ± SDs (Citation: Ref. [43])

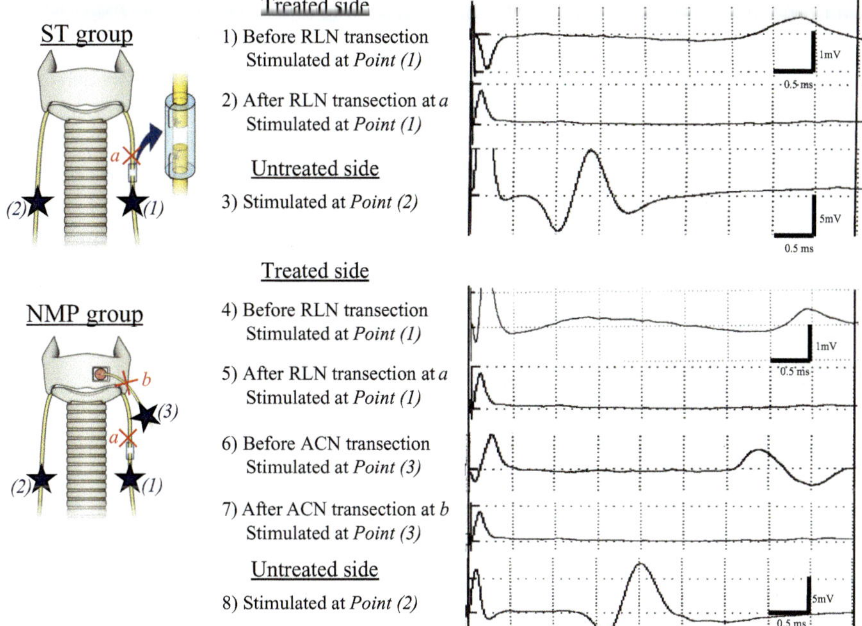

Fig. 3.46   Representative evoked electromyographic potentials in the silicone tube (*ST*) and NMP groups. *RLN* Recurrent laryngeal nerve, *ACN* ansa cervicalis nerve (Modified from Ref. [43])

3.3.4.5 Dual Innervation of the TA Muscle

In rats of the ST model, the number of NMJs was greater than that in the DNV model. Individual muscle fiber size was significantly greater in the ST than in the DNV model, but the vocal fold on the treated side remained immobile. Reinnervation by the RLN was proven by the presence of an evoked EMG response. Such findings suggest that the ST model simulates clinical cases of UVFP in whom partial RLN reinnervation occurs in the absence of vocal fold motion. The NMP procedure performed on the rats at 5 weeks after placement of cut ends of RLN in a silicone tube was effective (compared to the ST model) in reducing atrophic changes in the TA muscle and increasing synapse formation, even in the presence of partial RLN innervation. In addition, the EMG data showed that TA compound action potentials were elicited by stimulating the proximal sides of both the transected RLN and the transferred ACN. Thus, partially innervated TA muscle as a whole can accommodate both foreign motor nerves (e.g., the ACN) and reinnervation from the original RLN.

Why then has it been reported that innervated muscle fibers do not accept innervation from a foreign nerve? [73] We propose that because TA muscle fibers of the ST group varied in size (Fig. 3.41), some muscle fibers were innervated, whereas others were not. Muscle fibers lacking innervation can accommodate regenerating nerve fibers from a foreign nerve. Thus, the TA muscle in NMP animals underwent dual innervation from the RLN and ACN, although each individual muscle fiber was innervated by either the RLN or the ACN (not both). Figure 3.47 is a schematic of this assumption. Therefore, it may be expected that the NMP procedure will be effective in clinical practice if used to treat a TA muscle that is partially innervated by the RLN or reinnervated via the RLN.

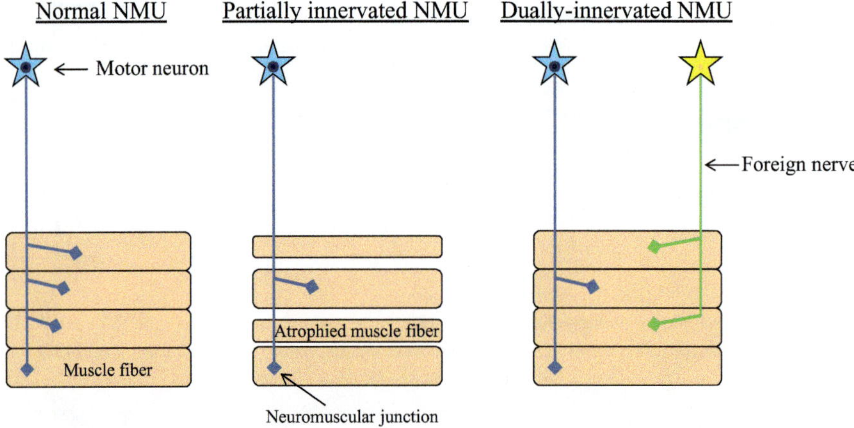

Fig. 3.47 Schematic representation of a neuromuscular unit (*NMU*) under normal, partially innervated, and dual-innervated conditions

References

1. Midrio M. The denervated muscle: facts and hypotheses. A historical review. Eur J Appl Physiol. 2006;98:1–21.
2. Schmalbruch H, Al-Amood WS, Lewis DM. Morphology of long-term denervated rat soleus muscle and the effect of chronic electrical stimulation. J Physiol. 1991;441:243–56.
3. Viguie CA, Lu DX, Huang SK, et al. Quantitative study of the effects of long-term denervation on the extensor digitorum longus muscle of the rat. Anat Rec. 1997;248:346–54.
4. Shindo ML, Herzon GD, Hanson DG, Cain DJ, Sahgal V. Effects of denervation on laryngeal muscles: a canine model. Laryngoscope. 1992;102:663–9.
5. Shinners MJ, Goding GS, McLoon LK. Effect of recurrent laryngeal nerve section on the laryngeal muscles of adult rabbits. Otolaryngol Head Neck Surg. 2006;134:413–8.
6. Winlow W, Usherwood PN. Ultrastructural studies of normal and degenerating mouse neuromuscular junctions. J Neurocytol. 1975;4:377–94.
7. Frank E, Gautvik K, Sommerschild H. Persistence of junctional acetylcholine receptors following denervation. Cold Spring Harb Symp Quant Biol. 1976;40:275–81.
8. Andreose JS, Fumagalli G, Lomo T. Number of junctional acetylcholine receptors: control by neural and muscular influence in the rat. J Physiol. 1995;483:397–406.
9. Portillo F, Pasaro R. Location of motoneurons supplying the intrinsic laryngeal muscles of rats. Horseradish peroxidase and fluorescence double-labeling study. Brain Behav Evol. 1988;32:220–5.
10. Lobera B, Pasaro R, Gonzalez-Baron S, Delgado-Garcia JM. A morphological study of ambiguus nucleus motoneurons innervating the laryngeal muscles in the rat and cat. Neurosci Lett. 1981;23:125–30.
11. Yoshida Y, Yatake K, Tanaka Y, et al. Morphological observation of laryngeal motoneurons by means of cholera toxin B subunit tracing technique. Acta Otolaryngol. 1998;118 Suppl 539:98–105.
12. Komori M. Effects of neurotrophic factors on regeneration of denervated recurrent laryngeal nerve in the rat. Pract Otorhinolaryngol. 1999;92:677–86. (in Japanese)
13. Sanuki T, Yumoto E, Komori M, Hyodo M. Expression of fibroblast growth factor-2 in the nucleus ambiguus following recurrent laryngeal nerve injury in the rat. Laryngoscope. 2000;110:2128–34.
14. Sunderland S. A classification of peripheral nerve injuries producing loss of function. Brain. 1951;74:491–516.
15. Huber K, Meisinger C, Grotiie C. Expression of fibroblast growth factor-2 in hypoglossal motoneurons is stimulated by peripheral nerve injury. J Comp Neurol. 1997;382:189–98.
16. Fujimoto E, Mizoguchi A, Hanada K, Yajima M, Ide C. Basic fibroblast growth factor promotes extension of regenerating axons of peripheral nerve. In vivo experiments using a Schwann cell basal lamina tube model. J Neurocytol. 1997;26:511–28.
17. Kobayashi J, Mackinnon SE, Watanabe O, Ball DJ, Gu XM, Hunter DA, Kuzon Jr WM. The effect of duration of muscle denervation on functional recovery in the rat model. Muscle Nerve. 1997;20:858–66.
18. Johns MM, Urbanchek M, Chepeha DB, Kuzon Jr WM, Hogikyan ND. Thyroarytenoid muscle maintains normal contractile force in chronic vocal fold immobility. Laryngoscope. 2001;111:2152–6.
19. Kirchner JA. Atrophy of laryngeal muscles in vagal paralysis. Laryngoscope. 1966;76:1753–65.
20. Kirchner JA. Intrathoracic injury to the motor nerve supply of the larynx. Acta Otolaryngol. 1977;83:163–9.
21. Kawakita S, Aibara R, Kawamura Y, Yumoto E, Desaki J. Motor innervation of the guinea pig interarytenoid muscle: reinnervation process following unilateral denervation. Laryngoscope. 1998;108:398–402.

22. Gacek M, Gacek RR. Cricoarytenoid joint mobility after chronic vocal cord paralysis. Laryngoscope. 1996;106:1528–30.
23. Müller A, Paulsen FP. Impact of vocal cord paralysis on cricoarytenoid joint. Ann Otol Rhinol Laryngol. 2002;111:896–901.
24. Brown MC, Holland RL, Hopkins WG. Motor nerve sprouting. Ann Rev Neurosci. 1981;4:17–42.
25. Miyauchi A, Matsusaka K, Kihara M, Matsuzuka F, Hirai K, Yokozawa T, Kobayashi A, Kuma K. The role of ansa-to-recurrent laryngeal nerve anastomosis in operations for thyroid cancer. Eur J Surg. 1998;164:927–33.
26. Miyauchi A, Inoue H, Tomoda C, Fukushima M, Kihara M, Higashiyama T, Takamura Y, Ito Y, Kobayashi K, Miya A. Improvement in phonation after reconstruction of the recurrent laryngeal nerve in patients with thyroid cancer invading the nerve. Surgery. 2009;146:1056–62.
27. Yumoto E, Sanuki T, Kumai Y. Immediate recurrent laryngeal nerve reconstruction and vocal outcome. Laryngoscope. 2006;116:1657–61.
28. Sanuki T, Yumoto E, Minoda R, Kodama N. The role of immediate recurrent laryngeal nerve reconstruction for thyroid cancer surgery. J Oncol. 2010;2010:846235.
29. Aitken JT. Problems of reinnervation of muscle. Prog Brain Res. 1965;14:232–62.
30. Anzil AP, Wernig A. Muscle fibre loss and reinnervation after long-term denervation. J Neurocytol. 1989;18:833–45.
31. Su WF, Hsu YD, Chen HC, Sheng H. Laryngeal reinnervation by ansa cervicalis nerve implantation for unilateral vocal cord paralysis in humans. J Am Coll Surg. 2007;204:64–72.
32. Frey M, Gruber H, Holle J, Freilinger G. An experimental comparison of the different kinds of muscle reinnervation: nerve suture, nerve implantation, and muscular neurotization. Plast Reconstr Surg. 1982;69:656–67.
33. Cedars MG, Miller TA. A review of free muscle grafting. Plast Reconstr Surg. 1984;74:712–20.
34. Hogikyan ND, Johns MM, Kileny PR, Urbanchek M, Carroll WR, Kuzon WM. Motion-specific laryngeal reinnervation using muscle-nerve-muscle neurotization. Ann Otol Rhinol Laryngol. 2001;110:801–10.
35. Debnath I, Rich JT, Paniello RC. Intrinsic laryngeal muscle reinnervation using muscle-nerve-muscle technique. Ann Otol Rhinol Laryngol. 2008;117:382–8.
36. Sato F, Ogura JH. Functional restoration for recurrent laryngeal paralysis: an experimental study. Laryngoscope. 1978;88:855–71.
37. Meikle D, Trachy RE, Cummings CW. Reinnervation of skeletal muscle: a comparison of nerve implantation with neuromuscular pedicle transfer in an animal model. Ann Otol Rhinol Laryngol. 1987;96:152–7.
38. Tucker HM. Reinnervation of the unilaterally paralyzed larynx. Ann Otol Rhinol Laryngol. 1977;86:789–94.
39. Tucker HM, Rusnov M. Laryngeal reinnervation for unilateral vocal cord paralysis: long-term results. Ann Otol Rhinol Laryngol. 1981;90:457–9.
40. May M, Beery Q. Muscle-nerve pedicle laryngeal reinnervation. Laryngoscope. 1986;96:1196–200.
41. Zheng H, Zhou S, Chen S, Li Z, Cuan Y. An experimental comparison of different kinds of laryngeal muscle reinnervation. Otolaryngol Head Neck Surg. 1998;119:540–7.
42. Sayers H, Tonge DA. A study of factors influencing synapse formation by a foreign nerve in skeletal muscleof *Rana pipiens*. J Physiol Lond. 1986;375:449–60.
43. Aoyama T, Kumai Y, Yumoto E, Ito T, Miyamaru S, Sanuki T. Effects of nerve-muscle pedicle on the rat immobile vocal fold in the presence of partial innervations. Ann Otol Rhinol Laryngol. 2010;119:823–9.
44. Dupont-Versteegden EE, Houle JD, Gureley CM, Peterson CA. Early changes in the muscle fiber size and gene expression in response to spinal cord transection and exercise. Am J Physiol. 1998;275:1124–33.

45. Keilhoff G, Fansa H. Successful intramuscular neurotization is dependent on the denervation period. A histomorphological study of the gracilis muscle in the rats. Muscle Nerve. 2005;31:221–8.
46. Kumai Y, Ito T, Matsukawa A, Yumoto E. Effects of denervation on neuromuscular junctions in the thyroarytenoid muscle. Laryngoscope. 2005;115:1869–72.
47. Widenmann B, Frank WW. Identification and localization of synaptophysin, an integral membrane glycoprotein of Mr 38,000 characteristic of presynaptic vesicles. Cell. 1985;41:1017–28.
48. Anderson MJ, Cohen MW. Fluorescent staining of acetylcholine receptors in vertebrate skeletal muscle. J Physiol. 1974;237:385–400.
49. Miyamaru S, Kumai Y, Ito T, Yumoto E. Effects of long-term denervation on the rat thyroarytenoid muscle. Laryngoscope. 2008;118:1318–23.
50. Nomoto M, Yoshihara T, Kanda T, Kaneko T. Synapse formation by autonomic nerves in the previously denervated neuromuscular junctions of the feline intrinsic muscles. Brain Res. 1991;539:276–86.
51. Dedo HH, Ogura JH. Vocal cord electromyography in the dog. Laryngoscope. 1965;75:201–11.
52. Tucker HM. Long-term results of nerve-muscle pedicle reinnervation for laryngeal paralysis. Ann Otol Rhinol Laryngol. 1989;98:674–6.
53. Hengener AS, Tucker HM. Restoration of abduction in the paralyzed canine vocal fold. Arch Otolaryngol. 1973;97:247–50.
54. Lyons RM, Tucker HM. Delayed restoration of abduction in the paralyzed canine larynx. Arch Otolaryngol. 1974;100:176–9.
55. Anonsen CK, Patterson HC, Trachy RE, Gordon AM, Cummings CW. Reinnervation of skeletal muscle with a neuromuscular pedicle. Otolaryngol Head Neck Surg. 1985;93:48–57.
56. Fata JJ, Malmgren LT, Gacek RR, Dum R, Woo P. Histochemical study of posterior cricoarytenoid muscle reinnervation by a nerve-muscle pedicle in the cat. Ann Otol Rhinol Laryngol. 1987;96:479–87.
57. Rice DH, Owens O, Burstein F, Verity A. The nerve-muscle pedicle. Arch Otolaryngol. 1983;109:233–4.
58. Crumley RL. Experiments in laryngeal reinnervation. Laryngoscope. 1982;92 Suppl 3:1–27.
59. Kumai Y, Ito T, Udaka N, Yumoto E. Effects of a nerve-muscle pedicle on the denervated rat thyroarytenoid muscle. Laryngoscope. 2006;116:1027–32.
60. Windidch A, Gundersen K, Szabolcs M, Gruber H, Lømo T. Fast to slow transformation of denervated and electrically stimulated rat muscle. J Physiol. 1998;510:623–32.
61. Sterne GD, Coulton GR, Brown RA, et al. Neurotrophin-3-enhanced nerve regeneration selectively improves recovery of muscle fibers expressing myosin heavy chains 2b. J Cell Biol. 1997;139:709–15.
62. Miyamaru S, Kumai Y, Ito T, Sanuki T, Yumoto E. Nerve-muscle pedicle implantation facilitates re-innervation of long-term denervated thyroarytenoid muscle in rats. Acta Otolaryngol. 2009;129:1486–92.
63. Nguyen QT, Sanes JR, Lichtman JW. Pre-existing pathways promote precise projection patterns. Nat Neurosci. 2002;5:861–7.
64. Bader D. Reinnervation of motor endplate-containing and motor endplate-less muscle grafts. Dev Biol. 1980;77:315–27.
65. Hawke TJ, Garry DJ. Myogenic satellite cells: physiology to molecular biology. J Appl Physiol. 2001;91:534–51.
66. Miyamaru S, Kumai Y, Minoda R, Yumoto E. Nerve-muscle pedicle implantation in the denervated thyroarytenoid muscle of aged rats. Acta Otolaryngol. 2012;132:210–7.
67. Connor NP, Suzuki T, Lee K, Sewall GK, Heisey DM. Neuromuscular junction changes in aged rat thyroarytenoid muscle. Ann Otol Rhinol Laryngol. 2002;111:579–86.
68. McMullen CA, Andrade FH. Functional and morphological evidence of age-related denervation in rat laryngeal muscles. J Gerontol A Biol Sci Med Sci. 2009;64:435–42.

69. Suzuki T, Connor NP, Lee K, Bless DM, Ford CN, Inagi K. Age-related alterations in myosin heavy chain isoforms in rat intrinsic laryngeal muscle. Ann Otol Rhinol Laryngol. 2002;111:962–7.
70. McMullen CA, Andrade FH. Contractile dysfunction and altered metabolic profile of the aging rat thyroarytenoid muscle. J Appl Physiol. 2006;100:602–8.
71. Malmgren LT, Jones CE, Bookman LM. Muscle fiber and satellite cell apoptosis in the aging human thyroarytenoid muscle: a stereological study with confocal laser scanning microscopy. Otolaryngol Head Neck Surg. 2001;125:34–9.
72. Mark RF. Selective innervation of muscle. Br Med Bull. 1974;30:122–5.
73. Kumai Y, Aoyama T, Nishimoto K, Sanuki T, Minoda R, Yumoto E. Recurrent laryngeal nerve regeneration through a silicone tube produces reinnervation without vocal fold mobility in rats. Ann Otol Rhinol Laryngol. 2013;122:49–53.
74. Crumley R. Laryngeal synkinesis revisited. Ann Otol Rhinol Laryngol. 2000;109:365–71.

Chapter 4
Diagnosis of Paralytic Dysphonia
and Its Clinical Characteristics

Abstract Three-dimensional (3D) computed tomography is used to assess the 3D configuration of the laryngeal lumen. We propose a novel classification of 3D glottal configuration, in which the thickness of the affected vocal fold during phonation is the key determinant. In the type A configuration, the thickness is nearly equal to that of the unaffected vocal fold. In the type B situation, the affected fold is thinner than the other fold during both phonation and inhalation. In the type C condition, the affected fold is thinner than the other during phonation but, paradoxically, exhibits adduction and an increase in thickness during inhalation. Vocal function in patients with the type A configuration is significantly better than in those with type B or C configurations, whereas no significant difference in vocal function is evident between patients with configurations of types B and C. Over-adduction of the unaffected vocal fold may not compensate for vocal function. Further studies are necessary to associate glottal configuration types with reinnervation patterns evident upon electromyographic analysis and to determine why some patients with unilateral vocal fold paralysis exhibit over-adduction of the unaffected fold during phonation whereas others do not, despite the presence of a posterior glottal gap.

Keywords Three-dimensional computed tomography • Glottal configuration • Vocal function • Over-adduction of the unaffected vocal fold • Electromyographic recruitment

4.1 Introduction

The presence of unilateral vocal fold paralysis (UVFP), determined by videoendoscopy of the larynx,   has prompted a search for the underlying cause. The investigations routinely performed at the author's institution are shown in Fig. 2.1. When the cause was established, treatment followed. Later, the symptoms of VFP[1] were addressed. This chapter will deal with the diagnostic battery available for patients

---

[1] Breathy dysphonia and poor swallowing in patients with unilateral VFP and inspiratory dyspnea in those with bilateral VFP

© Springer Japan 2015

E. Yumoto, *Pathophysiology and Surgical Treatment of Unilateral Vocal Fold Paralysis*, DOI 10.1007/978-4-431-55354-0_4

with breathy dysphonia caused by UVFP. In addition, the clinical characteristics of UVFP studied at the author's institution will be described.

4.2   The Vocal Function Test Battery

Voice production is a complex process that involves appropriate coordination of many organs. Respiratory organs provide airflow, which is the driving force behind vocal fold vibration. The vocal fold plays an essential role in the production of glottal sound. Such sound is resonated as the sound traverses the vocal tract and is finally radiated through the mouth and nose. In this book, the laryngeal aspects of sound production are discussed; it will be assumed that the respiratory and articulatory systems are functioning well.

Figure 4.1 shows a flow chart of the vocal function tests in the test battery administered to UVFP patients in the author's institution. First, history taking explores the patient's occupation and hobbies, which may be associated with vocal usage. Also, the patient's attitude to breathy dysphonia is subjectively assessed using a voice handicap index (VHI [1], VHI-10 [2]) and a voice-related quality-of-life (V-RQOL) instrument [3]. Videostroboscopy is the most useful tool for observation of vocal fold vibration. Figure 4.2 shows the items that must be evaluated videostroboscopically. Although the technique does not permit analysis of every vibratory cycle, average patterns of vocal fold vibration can be observed. However, if the voice is severely breathy, strobe

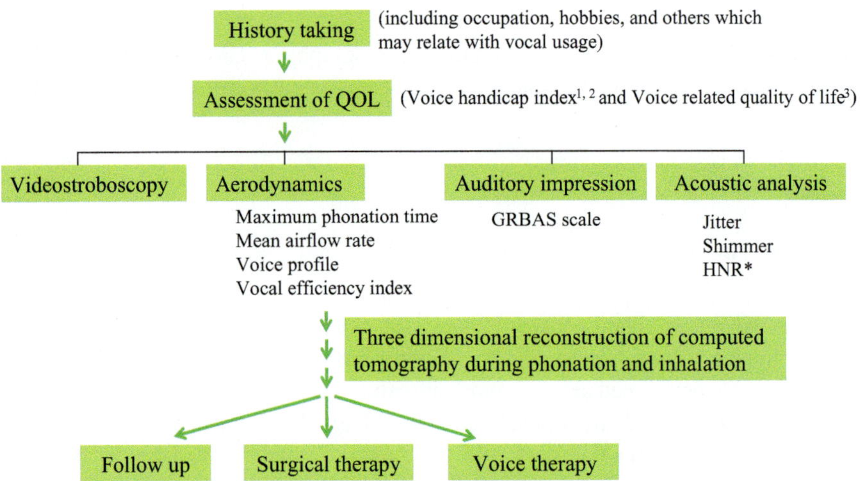

*HNR: Harmonics-to-noise ratio, An acoustic energy ratio of harmonic component to noise component in a sustained vowel /a/. [58]–[60]

Fig. 4.1 Flow chart showing how to administer a vocal function test battery to patients with unilateral vocal fold paralysis

(1) Parameters regarding vocal fold vibration

    ✓ Glottal gap: presence, size, and location
    ✓ Mucosal wave: regularity, symmetry
    ✓ Deviation of glottal axis towards the affected side
    ✓ Supraglottal constriction: over-adduction of the ventricular fold and anterior-posterior shortening

(2) Parameters regarding the vocal fold on the affected side

    ✓ Mobility and flaccidity
    ✓ Synkinesis
    ✓ Anterior tilt of the arytenoid mound

(3) Parameters regarding the vocal fold on the unaffected side

    ✓ Mobility
    ✓ Over-adduction

Fig. 4.2 Parameters to be evaluated during videostroboscopy

illumination is not synchronized and irregular mucosal movement is observed. Furthermore, in-depth information such as differences in the thicknesses of and the vertical distance between the vocal folds is not readily obtainable using this method.

The aerodynamics of voice production involve differences between subglottal and supraglottal pressures. Imperfect closure of the glottis during phonation by UVFP patients decreases glottal resistance, elevates supraglottal pressure, and reduces the vocal efficiency index. [4] Such glottal insufficiency is reflected by an increase in the mean airflow rate (MFR) and a reduction in maximum phonation time (MPT), as measured via sustained vowel phonation at a comfortable pitch and loudness. A voice profile is also obtained to detect pathological changes in the voice for which other parameters remain within normal ranges. Titze [5] originally defined a voice range profile as a comparison of vocal intensity versus fundamental frequency (F_0). The voice profile most commonly used in Japan displays not only vocal intensity versus F_0 but also a combination of three parameters: intensity, F_0, and MFR. [6] The auditory impression of dysphonia is evaluated using the GRBAS scale, which is an acronym for grade overall, rough, breathy, asthenic, and strained [7]. Objective voice assessment evaluates acoustic parameters including jitter [8], shimmer [9], and the harmonics-to-noise ratio (HNR) [10].

4.3   Image Analysis of Unilateral Vocal Fold Paralysis

Videostroboscopy of the larynx cannot be used to assess differences in the thicknesses of and the vertical distance between the vocal folds. Hong and Jung [11], using stroboscopic images, evaluated the height of the affected fold compared to that of the unaffected fold based on the contact pattern of the vocal processes and the brightness of the vocal fold during phonation. It was found that the height of the affected fold was nearly equal to that of the unaffected fold when the affected fold was located at the midline. Furthermore, they reported that in half of UVFP patients in whom the affected fold was located off the midline, the affected fold was lower than the other. Upon analysis of stroboscopic images, Inagi et al. [12] found that UVFP patients exhibiting off-plane vocal fold closure during phonation developed hyperfunctionality (increased effort to compensate for the deficit). The cited authors stressed the importance of the shape of the subglottis and the glottal plane of closure, in determining convergence of the vocal fold during phonation. Gray et al. [13] also emphasized the importance of the infraglottal shape in terms of ease of phonation. Inagi et al. [12] suggested that radiographic techniques should be used to complement videostroboscopy to allow depth information to be obtained more readily.

Isshiki and Ishikawa [14] used conventional X-ray tomography to observe the laryngeal lumen during both phonation and inhalation in patients with UVFP. They found that the affected vocal fold was thinner than the healthy fold in 38 % of patients and that in 46 % of patients the affected vocal fold was higher during phonation. Although differences in the vertical thicknesses of and the distance between vocal folds were assessed, they failed to relate the findings with vocal function. Computed tomography (CT) and magnetic resonance imaging (MRI) have also been used to assess the persistence of fat injected into the vocal fold [15–17] and to help design the window position of and the implant size required for type I thyroplasty [18]. However, the authors of the cited reports did not investigate vocal fold configuration during phonation. Yumoto et al. [19, 20] were the first to successfully use a 3D CT endoscopic technique to assess the normal laryngeal structure and pathological changes in patients with laryngeal cancer, UVFP, and vocal fold atrophy. Laryngeal images viewed from both the oral and tracheal sides were obtained, as were two vertically split hemilaryngeal images. With the exception of images from the oral side, reconstructed images cannot be obtained via endoscopic observation. It was found that a combination of 3D endoscopic and coronal multiplanar reconstruction (MPR) imaging yielded more diagnostic information on patients with UVFP than did axial images alone, although scanning was performed during breath hold; the report was inconclusive in terms of vocal function. The later development of multi-slice helical CT allowed high-speed data acquisition without affecting the resolution of the final image. The associated short scan times permit the use of the method for observing laryngeal structures in 3D during both phonation and inhalation [21–23]. The details of how the larynx is scanned to produce 3D images will be described in the next section.

4.3.1 Three-Dimensional Computed Tomography (3D CT)

4.3.1.1 Production of 3D Endoscopic and Coronal MPR Images

Figure 4.3 shows the body position of and the task performed by a patient, the model used for scanning, the features thereof, the method used to detect the mucosal surface of the laryngeal lumen, and the images that are produced. Each subject is scanned

A. Body position of subject
    Supine
    Neck slightly extended to avoid overlapping the larynx with the mandible

B. Task of subject
    1. Sustain the vowel /a/ for 5 s. Loudness might be very small.
    2. Slow inhalation for 5 s.
    Practice the task before scanning.

C. Model utilized and scanning condition
    General Electric, Lightspeed VCT(CT with 64 detector-row)
    120kv, 200mA, slice thickness of 0.625mm, table speed of 53.7mm/s
    Subject is scanned starting from the hyoid bone caudally for 1.8 s.

D. Detection of mucosal surface and production of endoscopic and coronal MPR images
    Two voxels smaller than -100 Hounsfild units served as the surface of the laryngeal lumen.
    Views from the oral and tracheal sides and 2 vertically split hemilaryngeal images
    Coronal MPR images (1~2mm thickness, perpendicular to the glottal axis)

Fig. 4.3 Body position of, and task performed by, a subject; the model utilized for scanning; the setting thereof; the method used to examine the mucosal surface of the laryngeal lumen; and images produced with the aid of multi-slice helical computed tomography

during phonation and, after a short rest, during inhalation. Pre-scanning practice is necessary to enable satisfactory task performance. Axial images are generated at 1-mm intervals by overlapping each adjacent image by 0.5 mm, and the images are sent to a workstation together with voxel data. A volume-rendering technique is used in the 3D endoscopic mode. Supraglottal structures evident in the oral view are removed to enable visualization of the vocal folds when supraglottal constriction occurs [21–23].

The CT dose index (CTDi) is calculated to estimate the approximate radiation dose given during the laryngeal scan. The total CTDi value of scanning during both phonation and inhalation is 25.45 milliGray (mGy). This value was compared to those associated with the scanning of other regions of the head and neck. The CTDi values for the paranasal sinuses and temporal bone, based on the settings used at Kumamoto University Hospital, are 30.25 mGy and 63.57 mGy, respectively. A temporal bone scan requires the collection of thin slices (0.5 mm thick), and the CTDi is more than double that associated with a laryngeal scan. Although the CTDi is relatively low, care should nonetheless be taken when scanning the larynges of UVFP patients.

4.3.1.2   3D Endoscopic and Coronal MPR Images from Patients Exhibiting Normal Vocal Fold Movement

Figures 4.4 and 4.5 show endoscopic and coronal MPR images from a 55-year-old male exhibiting sulcus vocalis during both inhalation and phonation. His vocal fold movement was normal. Abduction of the vocal folds during inhalation and

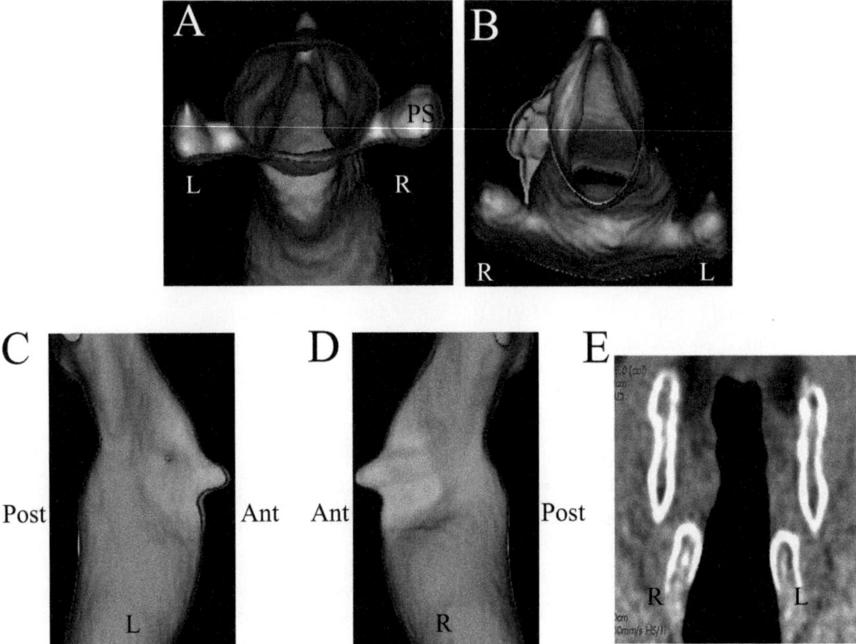

Fig. 4.4 CT endoscopic and coronal multiplanar reconstructed images of a 55-year-old male with sulcus vocalis and normal vocal fold movement, taken during inhalation. *A* Oral view, *B* Tracheal view, *C* Left hemilarynx viewed from the right, *D* Right hemilarynx viewed from the left, *R* Right, *L* Left, *Ant* Anterior, *Post* Posterior, *PS* Pyriform sinus (Citation: Ref. [22])

adduction during phonation were apparent on CT endoscopic images. During inhalation, the vocal folds were barely recognizable in either hemilaryngeal or coronal MPR images. The oral and tracheal views revealed that the vocal processes met at the midline during phonation. Coronal MPR images revealed that the vocal folds were symmetrical in terms of both thickness and the contours of the subglottic vault during phonation.

4.3.1.3   Representative Images of Unilateral Vocal Fold Paralysis

Figure 4.6 shows a representative UVFP case in whom the affected fold was as thick as the other fold and was located at the same level during phonation. The affected fold was directed medially, not superomedially, during phonation (Fig. 4.6, thin arrow), and remained adducted during inhalation (Fig. 4.6, thick arrow). A small glottal gap was evident between the vocal processes during phonation. These images suggest that synkinetic innervation was in play: the TA/LCA complex seemed to have received regenerated nerve fibers that originally innervated the posterior crico-arytenoid (PCA) muscle, because TA/LCA muscle contraction was evident during inhalation.

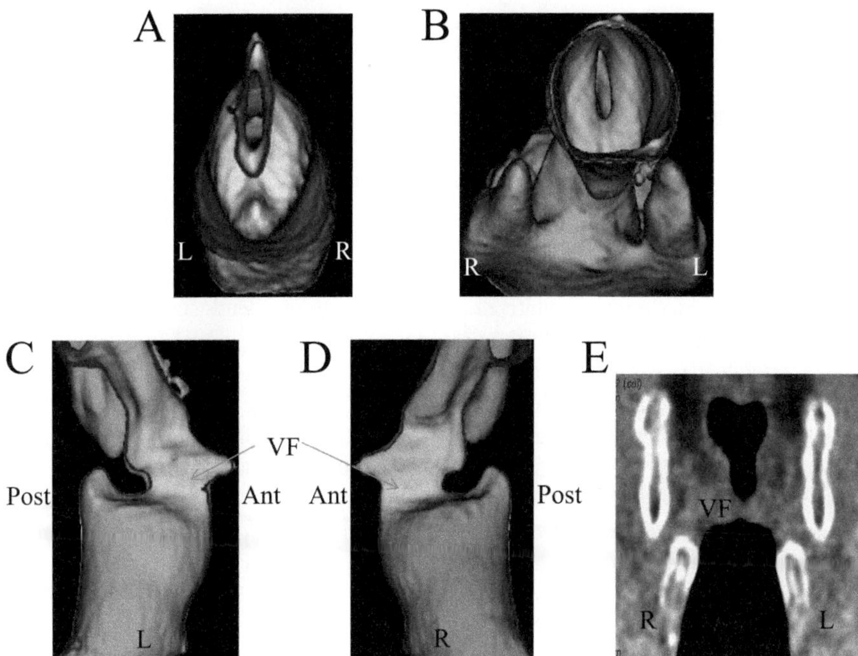

Fig. 4.5 CT endoscopic and coronal multiplanar reconstructed images taken during phonation of the subject mentioned in Fig. 4.4. *A* Oral view, *B* Tracheal view, *C* Left hemilarynx viewed from the right, *D* Right hemilarynx viewed from the left, *R* Right, *L* Left, *Ant* Anterior, *Post* Posterior, *VF* Vocal fold (Citation: Ref. [22])

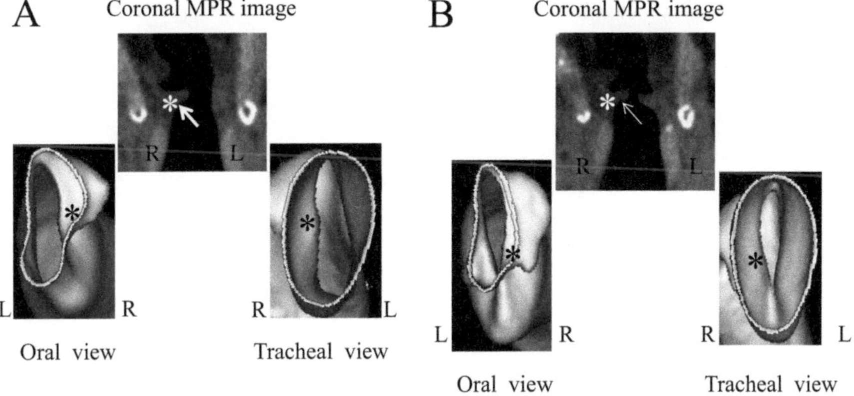

Fig. 4.6 CT endoscopic and coronal multiplanar reconstructed images of a 66-year-old female taken 7 months after onset of right vocal fold paralysis caused by thyroid cancer surgery. *A* Images taken during inhalation, *B* Images taken during phonation, *Affected side (Citation: Ref. [24])

Figure 4.7 shows a representative case in whom the affected fold was thinner and was located at a higher level than the healthy fold during phonation (thin arrow). Over-adduction of the healthy vocal fold was obvious during phonation. The affected fold remained thin and was directed superomedially during both phonation (thin arrow) and inhalation (thick arrow). A wide glottal gap between the vocal processes was evident during phonation, at which time the vocal folds could not be visualized videostroboscopically because of anterior-to-posterior constriction. Furthermore, the arytenoid portion of the healthy fold moved anteromedially during phonation, obstructing the view of the affected side (Fig. 4.8).

Figure 4.9 shows a representative case in whom the CT endoscopic and coronal MPR images were suggestive of the presence of paradoxical vocal fold movement. The affected fold was abducted during phonation and was barely recognizable in the coronal image. Furthermore, the fold was adducted (black arrows) and was thick during inhalation (thin white arrow). A wide glottal gap was evident between the vocal processes during phonation. Figure 4.10 shows videostroboscopic images taken during inhalation and phonation. The vocal process on the affected side could not be visualized during inhalation because of anterior tilting of the arytenoid portion. However, CT endoscopic and coronal images revealed that the affected fold was positioned near the midline during inhalation (Fig. 4.9, left). Thus, the location of the vocal fold could not be assessed in the absence of videostroboscopic visualization of the vocal process.

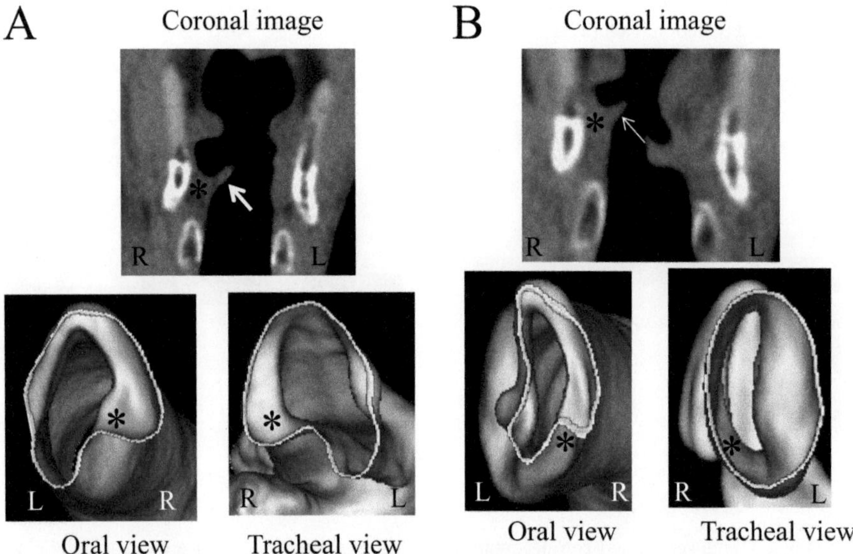

Fig. 4.7 CT endoscopic, coronal multiplanar reconstructed, and videostroboscopic images of a 68-year-old male taken 11 months after onset of right vocal fold paralysis caused by surgery to treat esophageal cancer. *A* Images taken during inhalation, *B* Images taken during phonation, *Affected side (Citation: Ref. [24])

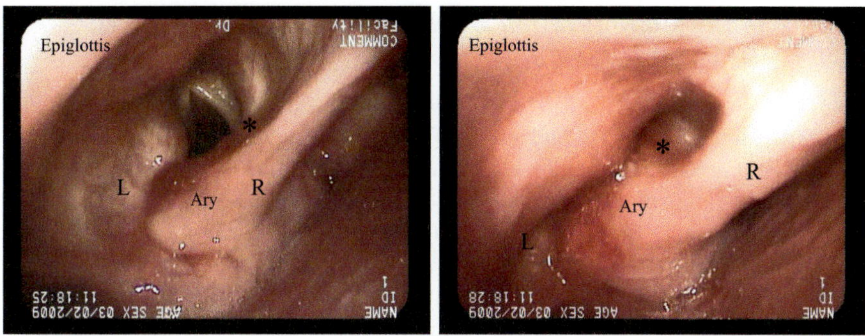

Fig. 4.8 Videostroboscopic images taken during inhalation (*left*) and phonation (*right*) by a 68 year-old male 11 months after onset of right vocal fold paralysis caused by surgery to treat esophageal cancer. This is the same subject as featured in Fig. 4.7, *Affected side, *Ary* Arytenoid portion on the affected side (Citation: Ref. [24])

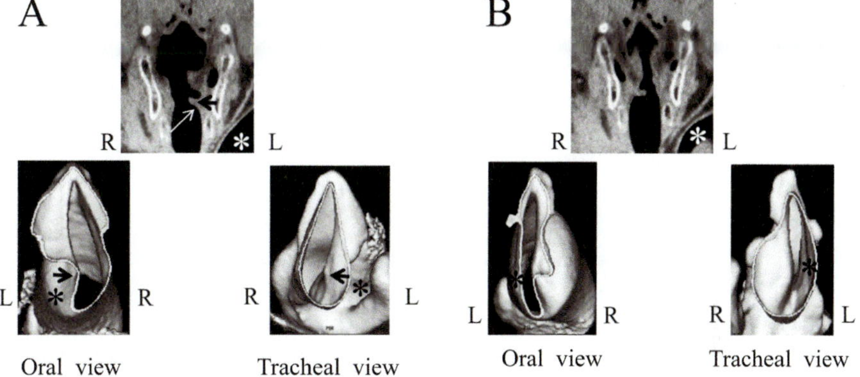

Fig. 4.9 CT endoscopic and coronal multiplanar reconstructed images of a 66-year-old male taken 13 months after onset of left vocal fold paralysis caused by surgery to treat thyroid cancer. *A* Images taken during inhalation, *B* Images taken during phonation, *Affected side (Citation: Ref. [24])

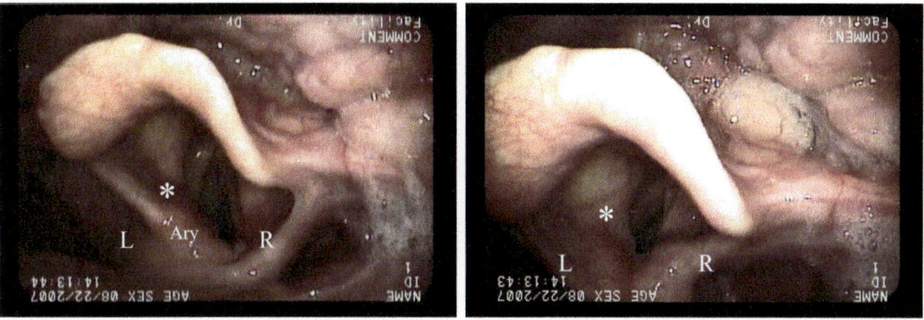

Fig. 4.10 Videostroboscopic images taken during inhalation (*left*) and phonation (*right*) of a 66-year-old male 13 months after onset of left vocal fold paralysis caused by surgery to treat thyroid cancer. This is the same subject as featured in Fig. 4.9, *Affected side, *Ary* Arytenoid portion of the affected side

4.3.2   Glottal Configuration During Phonation and Vocal Function

Videostroboscopy is the standard means used to evaluate the vocal folds of patients with UVFP. Glottal configuration varies in such patients. However, determination of the 3D configuration of a unilaterally paralyzed larynx during phonation remains diagnostically challenging. Such an examination should establish the location of the affected fold, the presence or absence of fold flaccidity, and the extent of the glottal gap during phonation. However, supraglottal constriction, specifically over-adduction of the ventricular fold, anterior-to-posterior shortening of the glottis, and anterior tilting of the arytenoid portion, may occur during phonation. These factors prevent visualization of the entire larynx, especially the vocal process and posterior glottis. Furthermore, videostroboscopy cannot be used to evaluate differences in the thicknesses and vertical positions of the vocal folds. Such in-depth information is important when seeking to determine the extent of convergence of the vocal folds during phonation [12].

This section will describe the glottal configuration of UVFP patients based on the thicknesses and locations of the vocal folds during both phonation and inhalation, utilizing 3D CT imaging. We propose a novel classification of 3D glottal configuration, which features four grades, each of which is compared to the associated vocal functionality [24]. Such a classification may enhance our understanding of glottal configuration in UVFP patients in terms of vocal function.

4.3.2.1   Subjects, Evaluation of Glottal Configuration, and Assessment of Vocal Function

Fifty-nine consecutive patients with paralytic dysphonia, who had experienced UVFP onset more than 6 months prior, underwent 3D CT between February 2002 and January 2010. Of the 59 patients, 22 were excluded. The exclusion criteria were poor respiratory or swallowing function (which might interfere with sustained phonation) in eight patients, poor performance of the phonatory or inhalatory task during CT scanning in seven patients, intracranial lesions in four patients, a past history of phonosurgery in two patients, and unknown time of UVFP onset in one patient. Thus, 37 patients were included in the study. Table 4.1 summarizes the demographic characteristics thereof, and the causes of UVFP are listed in Table 4.2.

Table 4.1 Subject profiles

Gender	24 males, 13 females
Age	27–82 years (56.6 ± 15.0)
Affected side	Left: 26, right: 11
Period from onset to CT scanning[a]	6–480 months (51.8 ± 105.6), median value: 11.0

Citation: Ref. [24]
Mean ± standard deviation
[a]More than 20 years in four subjects

Table 4.2 Causes of unilateral vocal fold paralysis

Postoperative	Thyroid gland surgery	13
	Aortic aneurysm	9
	Mediastinum tumor	4
	Esophageal cancer	2
	Lung cancer	1
Idiopathic		3
Other[a]		5
Total		37

Citation: Ref. [24]

[a]Other causes include aortic arch aneurysm, mediastinal cancer, pulmonary tuberculosis, carotid artery aneurysm, and parapharyngeal tumor

Details of the method used for CT scanning and production of CT endoscopic and coronal MPR images are described in Sect. 4.3.1.1. Two experienced laryngologists (E.Y. and T.S.), who were blinded to patient data, evaluated all of the CT endoscopic and coronal MPR images displayed on a monitor. Differences in fold thicknesses, and the vertical and horizontal positions assumed during phonation and inhalation, were evaluated. Differences in vertical levels were assessed with the aid of coronal MPR images taken just anterior to the vocal process. It was specifically noted whether the affected fold was directed medially or superomedially during phonation. Furthermore, changes in glottal configuration suggestive of paradoxical movements were carefully observed; these included an increase in thickness, adduction of the affected fold during inhalation, and abduction during phonation.

Maximum phonation time (MPT) and mean airflow rate (MFR) during sustained phonation were measured using a phonation analyzer (SK-99; Nagashima, Tokyo, Japan) within 2 weeks before the day on which 3D CT scanning was performed. Each patient was asked to sustain the vowel "a" at a comfortable pitch and loudness, for as long as possible. Of two consecutive measurements taken, the larger value was included in analysis. The data were compared to the glottal configuration types that were identified via 3D CT image analysis. The unpaired t-test was used to explore the significance of differences in MPT and MFR among patients with various types of glottal configurations. Fisher's exact test was employed to examine the significance of differences in the vertical positions of affected vocal folds during phonation (StatView; SAS Institute, Cary, NC). A P value <0.05 was deemed to indicate statistical significance.

4.3.2.2   Evaluation of Glottal Configuration Based on 3D CT Images

The vocal folds on the affected sides of 32 (86.5 %) of the 37 subjects were thinner than those on the healthy sides during phonation. In 18 subjects (48.6 %), the affected vocal fold was located at a higher position during phonation (Table 4.3). Figures 4.6, 4.7, and 4.9 show the three different types of glottal configuration (described in Sect. 4.3.1.3).

Table 4.3 Numbers of subjects with regard to thickness and vertical position of the vocal fold on the affected side during phonation compared to those on the healthy side in the three types of glottal configuration

Glottal configuration type	Thickness			Vertical position	
	Thinner	Equal	Thicker	Higher	Equal
A (10)	5[a]	3	2	1	9[b]
B (12)	12	0	0	7	5
C (15)	15	0	0	10	5
Total	32	3	2	18	19

Citation: Ref. [24]
[a]Thickness of the affected vocal fold in these five subjects was slightly thinner than its mate
[b]The affected vocal fold in one subject was located at the lower level

Table 4.4 Numbers of subjects showing paradoxical movement of the vocal fold on the affected side in the three types of glottal configuration

Glottal configuration type	Thicker during inhalation	Abduction during phonation or adduction during inhalation
A (10)	0	0
B (12)	0	4
C (15)	6[a]	12[a]
Total	6	16

Citation: Ref. [24]
The numbers in parentheses show that of the subjects in each glottal configuration type
[a]Three subjects showed two kinds of paradoxical movement

Differentiation of abduction during phonation from adduction during inhalation was not feasible because only static 3D CT images were available for evaluation. An increase in subglottal pressure during phonation may push up the affected fold if that fold has reduced muscle tonus. Therefore, the numbers of subjects who exhibited abduction during phonation or adduction during inhalation are listed in Table 4.4. Because the vocal folds on the affected sides of three subjects exhibited both types of paradoxical movement, an increase in thickness during inhalation and abduction during phonation or adduction during inhalation, a total of 19 of 37 subjects exhibited either one or two paradoxical movements. Figure 4.9 shows a representative case. The affected fold was abducted during phonation and was barely recognizable in the coronal image. The affected fold was adducted (Fig. 4.9, black arrows) and became thick during inhalation (Fig. 4.9, thin white arrow). A wide glottal gap developed between the vocal processes during phonation. Figure 4.10 shows videostroboscopic images taken during inhalation (left) and phonation (right) of a 66-year-old male with left vocal fold paralysis (the same subject discussed in Fig. 4.9) exhibiting left-sided abduction on phonation.

Because achievement of glottal closure and a symmetrical configuration of the vocal folds are important in terms of voice production, the thickness of the affected vocal fold during phonation was considered to be the critical issue when deriving the new classification. In the type A configuration, the thickness of the affected fold during phonation is equal to, or slightly less than, that of the healthy vocal fold. In this type of configuration, the affected fold is directed medially, not superomedially, during phonation (Fig. 4.6, thin arrow). Only a small glottal gap was evident between the vocal processes during phonation. Subjects in whom the affected fold was thinner than the other during phonation were further classified into types B and C. In the type B configuration, the affected fold remained thin during both phonation and inhalation (Fig. 4.7) and was directed superomedially on phonation (Fig. 4.7, thin arrow). In the type C configuration, the presence of one or two paradoxical movements of the affected fold caused the fold to be directed medially, not superomedially, during inhalation (Fig. 4.9, thin white arrow), and the fold was barely recognizable in the coronal image (Fig. 4.9) during phonation. A prominent glottal gap was evident between the vocal processes during phonation in patients with type B or C glottal configuration (Figs. 4.7 and 4.9). Figure 4.11 shows a schematic representation of the laryngeal lumen of a normally innervated larynx and those of the three different types of unilaterally paralyzed larynges (types A, B, C).

Of the 37 subjects, 10 were assigned to type A, 12 to type B, and the remaining 15 to type C. Table 4.3 lists the numbers of subjects in terms of the thickness and vertical position of the affected fold during phonation compared to those of the healthy fold, who exhibited the three types of glottal configuration. The differences in the vertical position of the affected fold during phonation of patients of types A and B, and of types A and C, were significant (P = 0.0310 and P = 0.0119, respectively). Table 4.4 lists the numbers of subjects exhibiting paradoxical movement of the affected fold, by glottal configuration type.

Table 4.5 lists vocal function data (means ± standard deviations, SDs) with P values. Both the MPT and MFR in subjects with the type A glottal configuration were significantly better than in subjects of type B or C, whereas no significant difference in either MPT or MFR was apparent between type B and C subjects.

4.3.2.3   Significance of the Classification of Glottal Configuration

The present study is the first to classify the glottal configurations of UVFP patients, based on the thickness and location of the vocal folds during phonation and inhalation, utilizing 3D CT images. Such information may be useful in the clinical management of patients suffering from breathy dysphonia caused by UVFP. For example, when the glottal configuration is of type C, as shown in Fig. 4.9, the affected vocal fold is adducted during inhalation, but is abducted during phonation, in association with development of a prominent glottal gap. The vocal process is relatively easy to observe endoscopically during inhalation but is often difficult to evaluate during phonation because of supraglottal constriction. In such a case, medialization laryngoplasty might be considered an appropriate treatment, based on videostroboscopic data. However, medialization laryngoplasty alone would not be adequate and should be combined with arytenoid adduction to move the affected fold to the midline.

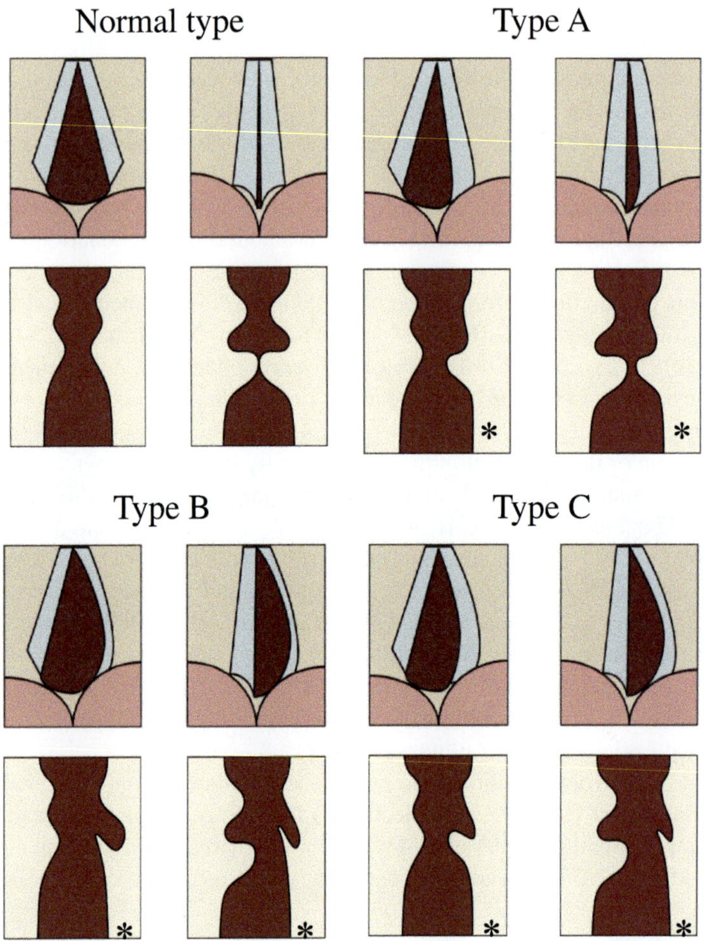

Fig. 4.11 Schematic representation of the laryngeal lumens of the normally innervated larynx and three different types of unilaterally paralyzed larynges (types A, B, and C). *Upper row* oral views, *Lower row* coronal images, *Left* inhalatory phase, *Right* phonatory phase, *Affected side (Citation: Ref. [24])

Furthermore, the thickness of the affected fold (compared to the healthy fold) and protrusion of the affected fold in the medial direction during phonation are used as primary classification criteria, because vocal function is expected to improve when the affected fold is as thick as, and located at the same level as, the healthy fold. The present study confirmed that vocal function was significantly better in patients with the type A configuration than in those with type B or C (Table 4.5). Because a denervated thin vocal fold is floppy, the fold is passively blown both upward and laterally as subglottal air pressure increases during phonation, and is drawn medially by the negative pressure associated with inhalation. Four subjects

Table 4.5 Vocal function in subjects of each glottal configuration type

Glottal configuration type	MPT (s)	MFR (mL/s)
A	9.04 ± 6.00 ⎤ P = 0.01255 ⎤	332.8 ± 204.7 ⎤ P = 0.0147 ⎤
B	4.50 ± 2.36 ⎦ ⎟ P = 0.0063	976.4 ± 735.6 ⎦ ⎟ P = 0.0050
C	4.02 ± 2.08 ⎦ NS ⎦	1019.3 ± 674.2 ⎦ NS ⎦

Citation: Ref. [24]
MPT maximum phonation time, *MFR* mean airflow rate

with such features were considered to have the type B configuration (Table 4.4). When increased air pressure pushes a floppy fold upward, such a fold becomes superomedially directed (Fig. 4.7, thin arrow). In contrast, the affected fold is directed medially, not superomedially, when adduction is associated with good muscle tonus (Figs. 4.6 and 4.9, white arrows). Such active adduction of the affected vocal fold is evident upon examination of morphological changes visible on CT endoscopic and coronal MPR images. An electromyographic (EMG) study is necessary to confirm the presence of active adduction.

Reinnervation patterns following development of UVFP can be divided into (1) low-level misdirected reinnervation resulting in normal or near-normal vocal fold movement; (2) reinnervation directed principally toward adductor muscle contraction during phonation and inhalation; (3) reinnervation directed principally toward adductor muscle contraction during inhalation, but not during phonation; (4) reinnervation directed principally toward abductor muscle contraction during both phonation and inhalation; (5) reinnervation directed principally toward abductor muscle contraction during phonation; and (6) barely detectable muscle contraction because of minimal reinnervation. The glottal configuration types proposed in the present study may be associated with such reinnervation patterns, as shown in Fig. 4.12. The type A glottal configuration is caused by reinnervation pattern (2). The type B configuration can be derived from reinnervation pattern (4), (5), or (6), and the type C configuration can be associated with reinnervation pattern (3) or (5). Thus, classification of glottal configuration based on 3D CT image analysis can be used to evaluate the reinnervation patterns of UVFP patients. Further electromyographic analysis is needed to associate the different glottal configurations with reinnervation patterns precisely.

4.3.3   Over-adduction of the Unaffected Vocal Fold During Phonation

In UVFP patients, adduction of the vocal fold on the unaffected side to a point over the midline (over-adduction) during phonation has historically been thought to improve vocal function by decreasing the size of the glottal gap [26]. Assuming

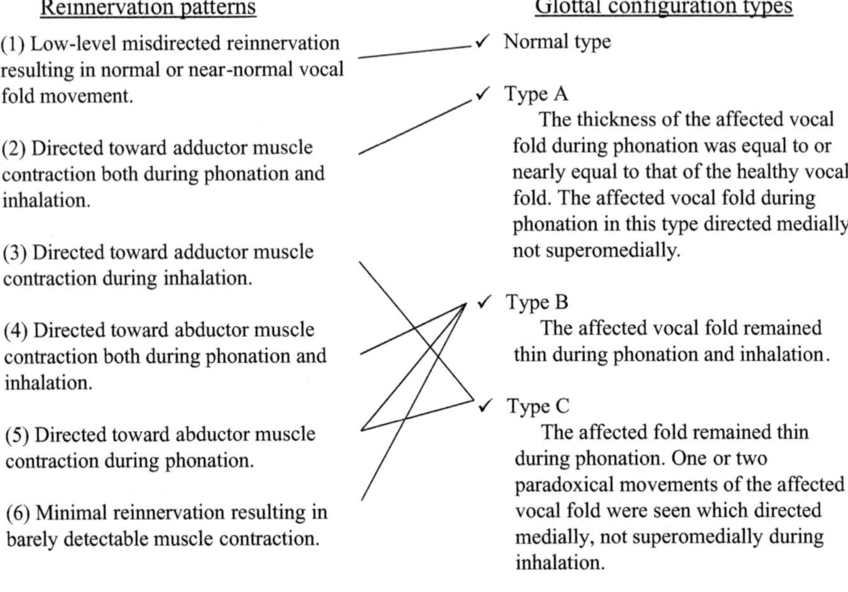

Fig. 4.12 Proposed relationships between possible reinnervation patterns and types of glottal configuration (Citation: Ref. [24])

that the cricoarytenoid joint in fact allows the vocal fold to adduct over the midline, a normal vocal fold may exhibit over-adduction during phonation in a UVFP patient whose affected vocal fold is located off the midline. In such a case, over-adduction of the unaffected vocal fold may occur spontaneously, but may not compensate vocal function. Thus, it remains to be clarified whether over-adduction of the unaffected vocal fold really plays a role in compensating vocal function in UVFP patients. This section will explore whether such over-adduction affects vocal function in patients with paralytic dysphonia. 3D CT endoscopic and coronal MPR images were used to explore the over-adduction of the vocal fold, the presence of a posterior glottal gap (i.e., a gap between the two vocal processes), and the differences in the vertical position and thickness of both vocal folds during phonation [25].

4.3.3.1　Subjects, Over-adduction, and Vocal Function

In total, 101 consecutive UVFP patients suffering from breathy dysphonia to varying extents, who underwent 3D CT examination during sustained phonation of the vowel "a," and during slow inhalation between August 1999 and November 2009, were included in the study. The exclusion criteria were paresis of the vocal fold, a past history of voice therapy or phonosurgical treatment, and an unknown time of UVFP onset. Videostroboscopy was performed on all patients on the day of their

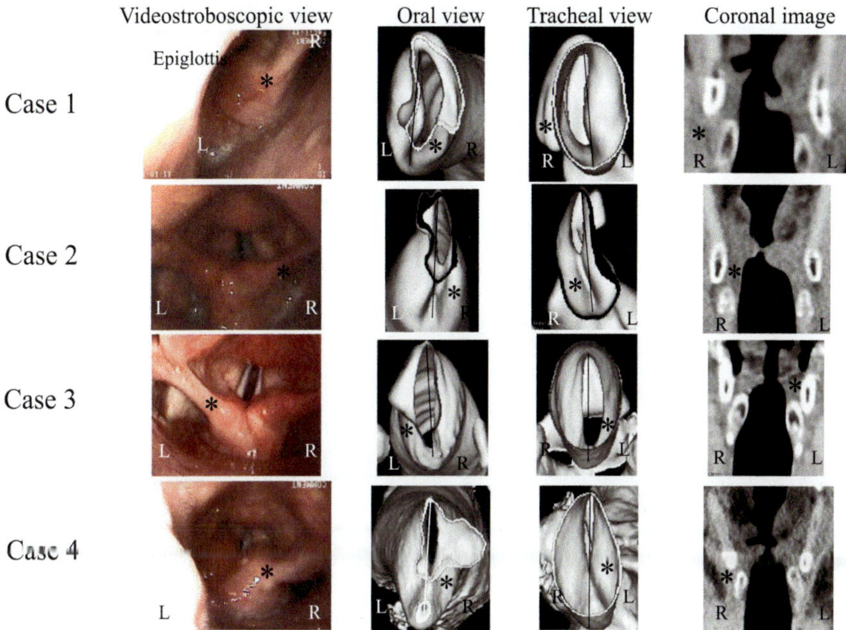

Fig. 4.13 Representative videostroboscopic and CT endoscopic images taken during phonation. *Case 1* Over-adduction of the unaffected fold with a posterior glottal gap, *Case 2* Over-adduction without a posterior glottal gap, *Case 3* No over-adduction with a posterior glottal gap. *Case 4* No over-adduction and no posterior glottal gap. *Lines* indicate the midline of the glottis. *L* Left, *R* Right, *Affected side (Citation: Ref. [25])

vocal function test. However, in some patients, visualization of the entire length of the vocal fold during phonation was not possible because of supraglottal constriction. Therefore, video recordings revealing the full extent of both folds during phonation were used to explore whether CT endoscopic images reflected the presence or absence of over-adduction of the unaffected vocal fold and a posterior glottal gap.

Two experienced laryngologists (E.Y. and T.S.) performed a single-blind evaluation of all of the CT endoscopic images. The glottal midline was drawn between the anterior commissure and the midpoint of the posterior wall of the glottis on CT endoscopic images from each patient (Fig. 4.13). Over-adduction was considered present when the vocal process of the unaffected fold was located beyond the theoretical midline of the glottis. Coronal images were used to evaluate differences in the thickness and vertical level of the vocal folds during phonation. MPT and MFR were measured as described in Sect. 4.3.2.1 and were chosen as useful indices of vocal function because the parameters reflect the amount of air escaping through the glottis during phonation.

Vocal function was compared between patients who did and did not exhibit over-adduction. Only data from subgroups of more than six patients were used in statistical analysis. The Mann–Whitney U test was employed to explore differences in

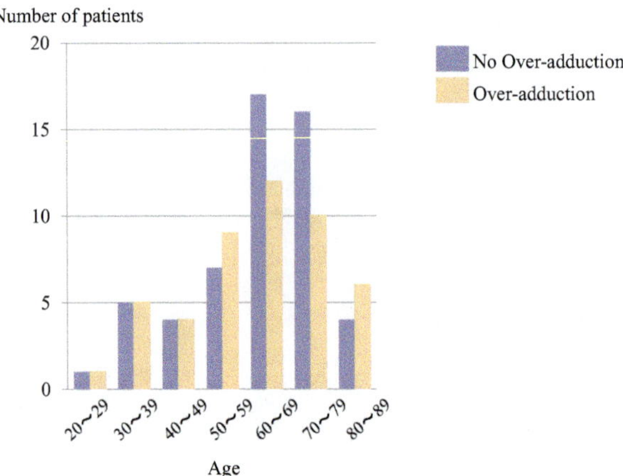

Fig. 4.14 Age distribution in terms of the presence of over-adduction of the unaffected vocal fold during phonation (Citation: Ref. [25])

MPT and MFR values among subgroups defined by evaluation of the 3D endoscopic and coronal images (StatView; SAS Institute, Cary, NC). In all analyses, $P < 0.05$ was deemed to indicate statistical significance.

4.3.3.2   Over-adduction and Clinical Features Thereof

Figures 4.14, 4.15, and 4.16 show the demographic characteristics of all 101 patients, including age distribution, cause of UVFP, and duration of UVFP from onset to the day of CT scanning. Patient age ranged from 27 to 84 years, and the mean and median ages were 61.6 years and 64 years, respectively. The cause of UVFP was divided into UVFP of iatrogenic origin or not. The duration of UVFP varied widely, ranging between 0.5 and 585 months, with a mean of 29.4 months and a median of 7.2 months.

The images in the upper two rows of Fig. 4.13 are representative CT endoscopic and videostroboscopic images, taken during phonation, of patients exhibiting over-adduction of the unaffected vocal fold, with or without a posterior glottal gap, respectively. The images in the lower two rows of Fig. 4.13 are representative CT endoscopic and videostroboscopic images, taken during phonation, of patients who did not exhibit over-adduction of the unaffected vocal fold, with or without a posterior glottal gap, respectively. As indicated in Fig. 4.13, the CT endoscopic images reflect the presence or absence of over-adduction of the unaffected vocal fold and a posterior glottal gap during phonation.

Of the 101 patients, over-adduction of the unaffected vocal fold was observed during phonation in 47 (46.5 %). Their MPT and MFR values were 4.9 ± 2.9 s (mean $\pm$ standard deviation) and 653 ± 504 mL/s, respectively. The remaining 54

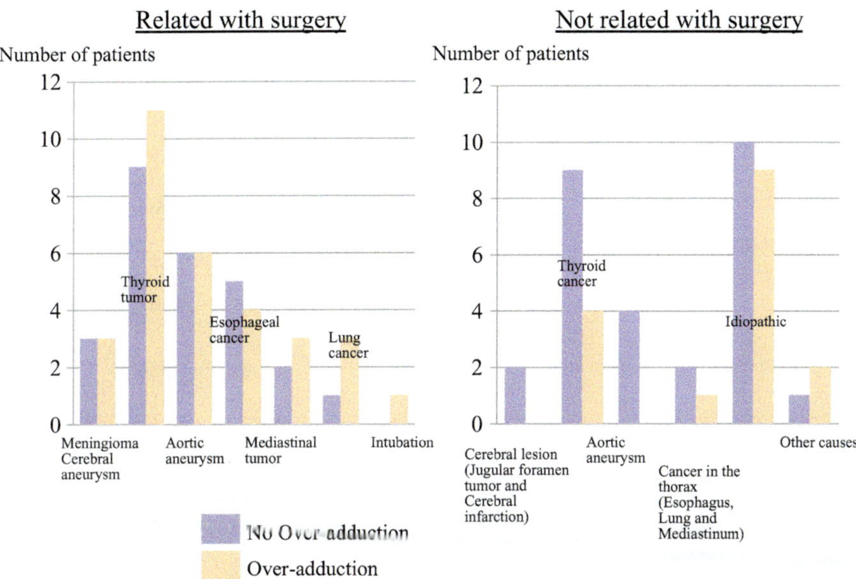

Fig. 4.15 Number of patients in each etiological class of unilateral vocal fold paralysis in terms of over-adduction of the unaffected vocal fold during phonation (Citation: Ref. [25])

Fig. 4.16 Effect of duration of unilateral vocal fold paralysis on the presence of over-adduction of the unaffected vocal fold during phonation (Citation: Ref. [25]

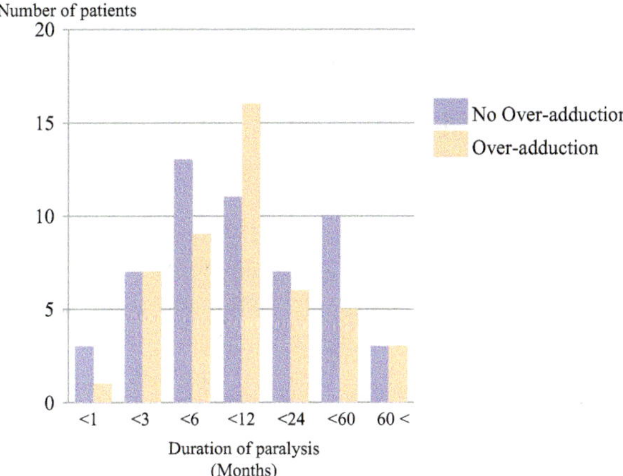

patients (53.5 %) did not exhibit over-adduction. Their MPT and MFR values were 4.7 ± 2.7 s and 574 ± 384 mL/s, respectively. Thus, no significant difference in either MPT or MFR was evident between the two groups ($P = 0.7080$ and 0.6954, respectively) (Table 4.6).

A posterior glottal gap was observed in 38 of the 47 patients (80.9 %) despite over-adduction of the unaffected vocal fold. The remaining nine patients did not

Table 4.6 P values in the comparison of vocal function between patients with over-adduction and those without over-adduction of the unaffected vocal fold during phonation

Subjects		Over-adduction	
		Present	Absent
All	Number of subjects	47	54
	MPT	NS (P=0.7080)	
	MFR	NS (P=0.6954)	
With posterior gap and higher position of the affected fold	Number of subjects	25	16
	MPT	NS (P=0.2136)	
	MFR	NS (P=0.3922)	
With posterior gap and no level difference between the folds	Number of subjects	12	25
	MPT	NS (P=0.3895)	
	MFR	NS (P=0.4172)	
With posterior gap and the affected fold being thinner	Number of subjects	30	38
	MPT	NS (P=0.4472)	
	MFR	NS (P=0.8919)	
No posterior gap and the affected fold being thinner	Number of subjects	8	9
	MPT	NS (P=0.8472)	
	MFR	NS (P=0.2110)	

Citation: Ref. [25]
MPT maximum phonation time, *MFR* mean airflow rate, *NS* not significant

have a posterior glottal gap (Table 4.7); 3D CT endoscopic images of eight of these nine patients indicated that the vocal folds overlapped, with the unaffected fold being situated below the affected fold (see the images in the second row of Fig. 4.13). A posterior glottal gap was observed in 43 of the 54 patients (79.6 %) in the absence of over-adduction of the unaffected vocal fold. No posterior glottal gap was evident in the 11 remaining patients (20.4 %) (Table 4.8); 3D CT endoscopic images of these 11 patients indicated that the vocal folds met at the midline without overlapping (see the images in the bottom row of Fig. 4.13).

Tables 4.7 and 4.8 list MPT and MFR values with reference to differences in the vertical position and thickness of the two vocal folds and the presence or absence of a posterior glottal gap. Vocal functions of patients exhibiting over-adduction are shown in Table 4.7, and those of patients who did not exhibit over-adduction are shown in Table 4.8. First, we compared vocal function between patients exhibiting over-adduction or not, during phonation, with reference to the presence of a posterior glottal gap and differences in the vertical position or thickness of the vocal folds. The P values are listed in Table 4.6; all are insignificant. Second, we compared patients exhibiting over-adduction of the unaffected vocal fold but no posterior gap, and those lacking over-adduction but who did have a posterior glottal gap, during phonation. The P values are listed in Table 4.9. When the affected fold was located at a higher position, the MPT was significantly longer in patients exhibiting over-adduction but lacking a posterior gap (6.3±2.7 s, see Table 4.7) than in those lacking over-adduction but with a posterior gap (3.2±1.2 s, see Table 4.8).

Table 4.7 Vocal function of patients with over-adduction of the unaffected vocal fold during phonation depending on the differences in vertical position and thickness between the vocal folds in relation with the presence or absence of a posterior glottal gap

			Posterior glottal gap	
			Present	Absent
	All subjects	Number of subjects	38	9
		MPT (s)	4.7±3.1 (3.9, 1.6–18.8)	5.8±2.4 (5.5, 2.8–10.2) P=0.1231
		MFR (mL/s)	661±506 (475, 85–2000)	615±528 (474, 148–1800) P=0.7456
Level difference (Higher side)	Paralyzed fold	Number of subjects	25	6
		MPT (s)	4.5±3.5 (3.4, 1.6–18.8)	6.3±2.7 (6.1, 2.8–10.2)
		MFR (mL/s)	784±545 (571, 131–2000)	487±350 (427, 148–1062)
	No difference	Number of subjects	12	3
		MPT (s)	5.1±1.9 (4.6, 2.7–8.5)	3.0, 5.5, 5.8
		MFR (mL/s)	438±332 (250, 85–932)	1,800, 275, 546
	Unaffected fold	Number of subjects	1	0
		MPT (s)	5.9	
		MFR (mL/s)	287	
Difference in thickness (Thinner side)	Paralyzed fold	Number of subjects	30	8
		MPT (s)	4.3±1.9 (3.7, 1.6–9.0)	5.5±2.4 (5.3, 2.8–10.2)
		MFR (mL/s)	688±540 (475, 85–2000)	673±534 (510, 148–1800)
	No difference	Number of subjects	7	0
		MPT (s)	6.3±5.9 (4.0, 2.7–18.8)	
		MFR (mL/s)	434±349 (725, 131–960)	
	Unaffected fold	Number of subjects	1	0
		MPT (s)	7.1	
		MFR (mL/s)	176	

Citation: Ref. [25]

MPT maximum phonation time, *MFR* mean airflow rate

Mean±SD, numbers in parenthesis: median value and range (minimum value and maximum value)

Difference in thickness could not be assessed in one patient without posterior glottal gap

Table 4.8 Vocal function of patients without over-adduction of the unaffected vocal fold during phonation depending on the differences in vertical position and thickness between the vocal folds in relation with the presence or absence of a posterior glottal gap

			Posterior glottal gap	
			Present	Absent
	All subjects	Number of subjects	43	11
		MPT (s)	4.1±2.0 (3.6, 1.3–9.6)	6.9±3.8 (5.6, 2.8–16.3)
		MFR (mL/s)	633±399 (546, 97–1800)	346±197 (313, 60–702)
Level difference (Higher side)	Paralyzed fold	Number of subjects	16	2
		MPT (s)	3.2±1.2 (3.2, 1.3–6.4)	2.8, 3.8
		MFR (mL/s)	867±440 (828, 205–1800)	702, 610
	No difference	Number of subjects	25	8
		MPT (s)	4.6±2.1 (4.0, 1.8–9.6)	7.7±4.1 (6.7, 4.0–16.3)
		MFR (mL/s)	492±291 (459, 97–1238)	291±138 (307, 60–523)
	Unaffected fold	Number of subjects	2	1
		MPT (s)	3.2, 7.8	7.8
		MFR (mL/s)	953, 103	159
Difference in thickness (Thinner side)	Paralyzed fold	Number of subjects	38	9
		MPT (s)	4.0±1.9 (3.5, 1.3–9.6)	6.5±4.2 (5.5, 2.8–16.3)
		MFR (mL/s)	617±375 (524, 97–1800)	366±209 (313, 60–702)
	No difference	Number of subjects	3	2
		MPT (s)	3.1, 4.3, 6.4	7.8, 9.5
		MFR (mL/s)	1365, 657, 205	159, 353
	Unaffected fold	Number of subjects	2	0
		MPT (s)	4.3, 8.7	
		MFR (mL/s)	1365, 176	

Citation: Ref. [25]
MPT maximum phonation time, *MFR* mean airflow rate
Mean±SD, numbers in parenthesis: median value and range (minimum value and maximum value)

Table 4.9 P values in the comparison of vocal function between patients with over-adduction of the unaffected vocal fold and no posterior gap and those without over-adduction and having posterior glottal gap during phonation

Subjects		Over-adduction: present Posterior gap: absent	Over-adduction: absent Posterior gap: present
All	Number of subjects	9	43
	MPT	NS (P=0.0514)	
	MFR	NS (P=0.7077)	
With the affected fold being in a higher position	Number of subjects	6	16
	MPT	P=0.0097	
	MFR	NS (P=0.0899)	
With the affected fold being thinner	Number of subjects	8	38
	MPT	NS (P=0.07458)	
	MFR	NS (P=0.9307)	

Citation: Ref. [25]
MPT maximum phonation time, *MFR* mean airflow rate, *NS* not significant

4.3.3.3   Does Over-adduction of the Unaffected Vocal Fold Really Compensate for Vocal Function?

In 1983, Yamada et al. [26] reported that only 41 (7.9 %) of 519 patients with UVFP exhibited over-adduction of the unaffected fold. Their retrospective evaluation of video recordings may have been difficult, because frequently, it is not possible to visualize completely both vocal folds during phonation. Thus, the reported incidence of over-adduction may have been an underestimate. However, Tanaka et al. [27] evaluated flexible endoscopic video recordings of 120 patients with UVFP and found over-adduction of the unaffected fold in 51 (42.5 %). When the vocal folds cannot be fiberscopically visualized because of supraglottal constriction, location of the arytenoid mound of the unaffected side at a position anterior to that on the paralyzed side was considered to indicate over-adduction of the unaffected fold. In our present study, over-adduction was evident in 47 (46.5 %) of 101 patients. Despite differences in the methods and criteria used by Tanaka et al. [27] and in the present study, the incidence rates are similar.

Our work does not support the proposition that over-adduction of the unaffected vocal fold contributes to better vocal function in patients with UVFP. Indeed, Tanaka et al. [27] found that vocal function (MPT and MFR data) was even worse in patients exhibiting over-adduction than in those lacking over-adduction. In the present study, 9 (19.1 %) of 47 patients exhibiting over-adduction did not have a posterior glottal gap, but vocal function in these 9 patients was no better than that of the remaining 38 patients exhibiting over-adduction with a posterior glottal gap (Table 4.7, P=0.1231 for MPT and P=0.7456 for MFR). In eight of the nine patients, the unaffected vocal fold was situated below the paralyzed fold (see images in the second row of Fig. 4.13). Such vertical disagreement in the absence of a posterior glottal gap creates an asymmetrical glottal configuration and glottal incompetence. However, no posterior glottal gap was noted in 11 (20.4 %) of 54 patients lacking over-adduction. Their vocal folds met at the midline without overlapping, and the thicknesses thereof were very similar (see images in the bottom row of Fig. 4.13.). These vocal folds were not mobile. Vocal function was significantly better in such patients than in the remaining 43 patients with posterior glottal gaps (Table 4.8, P=0.0068 for MPT and P=0.0192 for MFR). The most probable explanation is that the adductor muscles of patients without posterior glottal gaps may have undergone useful reinnervation, which led to muscle contraction during phonation despite no recovery of vocal fold movement. Electromyographic work is required to confirm this assumption.

Next, we compared patients exhibiting over-adduction but with no posterior glottal gap with those lacking over-adduction but with a glottal gap (Table 4.9). If it is assumed that over-adduction in patients with a posterior glottal gap represents an attempt to eliminate glottal insufficiency, over-adduction of the unaffected vocal fold could improve the MPT of patients in whom the affected fold is situated in a superior position. The MFR data showed such a tendency, but it was not significant (Table 4.9).

The question arises: Why does over-adduction occur in some patients but not others? Over-adduction of the unaffected vocal fold was not associated with patient age or the etiology or duration of UVFP. We did not perform follow-up scans because we sought to minimize radiation exposure. Thus, we do not know how long after UVFP onset over-adduction of the unaffected fold commenced. One patient with UVFP greater than 1 month in duration exhibited over-adduction of the unaffected vocal fold. However, among six patients with UVFP greater than 60 months in duration, over-adduction was absent in three patients. One possible explanation is that the articular surfaces of the cricoarytenoid joint vary among individuals. Although several authors have described the anatomy and movements of the cricoarytenoid joint [28, 29], possible adduction of the vocal fold over the midline was not evaluated. Gacek et al. [30] and Müller and Paulsen [31] histopathologically examined the cricoarytenoid joint on the paralyzed side, but not the unaffected side. Thus, whether the cricoarytenoid joint of some individuals is incapable of adduction over the midline remains to be determined.

In summary, over-adduction of the unaffected vocal fold may not compensate for vocal function in patients with UVFP. Further work is necessary to determine why some patients with UVFP exhibit over-adduction of the unaffected vocal fold during phonation, whereas others do not, despite the presence of a posterior glottal gap.

4.4 Electromyographic Recruitment, 3D Morphology of the Vocal Folds, and Vocal Function

The larynx rarely remains completely denervated or paralyzed after injury to the recurrent laryngeal nerve (RLN) (see Sect. 1.2 of Chap. 1). Laryngeal electromyography (LEMG) is useful for assessing the nature and extent of neurogenic pathology. LEMG can also aid in determining prognosis in terms of recovery of RLN function [32–39]. In this section, the laryngeal muscle activity of the TA/LCA complex will be examined with reference to differences in the height and thickness of the vocal folds during phonation, using aerodynamic measurements [40]. Coronal reconstructed images were obtained during phonation as described in Sect. 4.3.1.1. MPT and MFR were measured as described in Sect. 4.3.2.1.

4.4.1   Subjects and the LEMG Procedure

The subjects included 21 UVFP patients who were scheduled for laryngeal framework surgery (arytenoid adduction [AA] only, AA with type I thyroplasty, or AA with either ACN transfer or nerve–muscle pedicle flap implantation). All subjects underwent LEMG, aerodynamic analysis, and 3D CT examination between November 2005 and January 2010. Tables 4.10 and 4.11 show subject demographics and the causes of UVFP.

Each subject lay in a supine position with the neck extended using a shoulder roll. An EMG system (MEB-9200; Nihon Kohden, Tokyo, Japan) was used for evaluation; the filter settings were 20 Hz (low) and 10 kHz (high). EMG activities were recorded with a sweep speed of 10 ms and a gain of 200 mV per division. A second channel gathered data from a microphone timelocked to the EMG signal. Monopolar fine-wire platinum electrodes were placed percutaneously, through 23-gauge needles, into the TA/LCA muscle complex. The tips of the wires were

Table 4.10 Subject profiles

Gender	13 males, 8 females
Age	32–77 years (59.5 ± 14.4)
Affected side	Left: 16, right: 5
Period from onset to EMG	4–366 months (32.2 ± 789), median value: 9.0

Citation: Ref. [40]
Mean ± standard deviation

Table 4.11 Causes of unilateral vocal fold paralysis

Postoperative	Thyroid gland surgery	7
	Aortic aneurysm	5
	Esophageal cancer	3
	Mediastinum tumor	2
	Lung cancer	1
Idiopathic		1
Other	Lung tuberculosis	1
	Brain infarction	1
Total		21

Citation: Ref. [40]

bent backward to create a fishhook "barb" effect to hook the wire into the muscle as the insertion needle was withdrawn [41]. The TA/LCA muscle complex is typically located at a depth of 2 cm, and the location thereof was confirmed via video endoscopic monitoring and sustained vowel "i" phonation. A four-point scale was used to grade recruitment of EMG activity during phonation; this was the scale of Munin et al. [42] and Smith et al. [43] On this scale, 4+ represents no recruitment, 3+ greatly decreased recruitment, 2+ moderately decreased recruitment, and 1+ mildly decreased activity with an interference pattern that was less than full.

MU recruitment during LEMG and aerodynamic analysis was evaluated using Spearman's rank-correlation coefficients. Differences between LEMG findings, aerodynamic results, and coronal imaging data were analyzed using the Mann–Whitney U test. Statistical analysis was performed using StatView (SAS Institute, Cary, NC). In all analyses, $P < 0.05$ was deemed to indicate statistical significance.

4.4.2 LEMG Recruitment and Aerodynamic Analysis

Recruitment grade was 1+ for four patients, 2+ for five, 3+ for six, and 4+ for six patients. Nine of the 21 (42.9 %) patients with UVFP exhibited mildly or moderately decreased MU recruitment of the TA/LCA muscle complex during phonation. The LEMG and vocal functions are compared in Table 4.12. The recruitment grades of UVFP patients were negatively correlated with MPT ($rs = -0.51$, $P = 0.023$) and positively correlated with MFR ($rs = 0.48$, $P = 0.0322$).

4.4.3 LEMG Recruitment and 3D Morphology of the Vocal Folds

During phonation, the vocal folds on the affected sides of 19 (90.5 %) of the 21 subjects were thinner than the folds on the unaffected side. In 11 subjects (52.4 %), the affected vocal fold was higher than the unaffected fold during phonation

Table 4.12 Vocal function in subjects of each LEMG recruitments

MU recruitment	MPT (s)	MFR (mL/s)
1+ ($n = 4$)	4.95 ± 1.61	312.2 ± 156.7
2+ ($n = 5$)	5.82 ± 2.38	800.4 ± 566.4
3+ ($n = 6$)	3.78 ± 1.84	1066.6 ± 648.9
4+ ($n = 6$)	2.97 ± 1.23	791.8 ± 343.8

Citation: Ref. [40]
Mean ± standard deviation
MPT maximum phonation time, *MFR* mean airflow rate

Table 4.13 Recruitment of TA/LCA muscle complex with regard to thickness and vertical position of the vocal fold on the affected side compared to those on the unaffected side

	Thickness of vocal fold		Vertical position of vocal fold	
Recruitment	Thinner	Equal	Higher	Equal
1+ ($n=4$)	4	0	0	4
2+ ($n=5$)	4	1	0	5
3+ ($n=6$)	6	0	6	0
4+ ($n=6$)	5	1	5	1
Total	19	2	11	10

Citation: Ref. [40]

(Table 4.13). In all nine subjects with recruitment grades of 1+ and 2+, both folds were located at the same level. In 11 of 12 subjects with recruitment grades of 3+ and 4+, the affected folds lay superior to the unaffected folds. The vertical position of the affected fold was significantly associated with recruitment during phonation (P=0.0007).

In Sect. 4.3.2, we classified the glottal configurations of patients with UVFP into three types. Figure 4.12 shows a possible relationship between reinnervation patterns and the three proposed types of glottal configuration. Further work featuring simultaneous EMG recording of the activities of the TA/LCA complex and the PCA muscle is required to validate the assumptions made in Fig. 4.12.

References

1. Jacobson BH, Johnson A, Grywalski C, Silbergleit A, Jacobson G, Benninger MS, Newman CW. The voice handicap index (VHI): development and validation. Am J Speech Lang Pathol. 1997;6:66–70.
2. Rosen CA, Lee AS, Osborne J, Zullo T, Murry T. Development and validation of the voice handicap index-10. Laryngoscope. 2004;114:1549–56.
3. Hogikyan ND, Sethuraman G. Validation of an instrument to measure voice-related quality of life (V-RQOL). J Voice. 1999;13:557–69.
4. Isshiki N. Vocal efficiency index. In: Stevens KN, Hirano M, editors. Vocal fold physiology. Tokyo: University of Tokyo Press; 1981. p. 193–203.
5. Titze IR. Acoustic interpretation of the voice range profile (phonetogram). J Speech Hear Res. 1992;35:21–34.
6. Japan Society of Logopedics and Phoniatrics. Revised version: examination of voice. Tokyo: Ishiyakushuppan; 2009 (in Japanese).
7. Hirano M. Clinical examination of voice. Wien: Springer; 1981.
8. Liebermann P. Some acoustic measures of the fundamental periodicity of normal and pathologic larynges. J Acoust Soc Am. 1963;35:344–53.
9. Koike Y. Vowel amplitude modulations in patients with laryngeal diseases. J Acoust Soc Am. 1969;45:839–44.
10. Yumoto E, Gould WJ, Baer T. Harmonics-to-noise ratio as an index of the degree of hoarseness. J Acoust Soc Am. 1982;71:1544–50.

11. Hong KH, Jung S. Arytenoid appearance and vertical level difference between the paralyzed and innervated vocal cords. Laryngoscope. 2001;111:227–32.
12. Inagi K, Khidr AA, Ford CN, Bless DM, Heisey DM. Correlation between vocal functions and glottal measurements in patients with unilateral vocal fold paralysis. Laryngoscope. 1997;107:782–91.
13. Gray SD, Bielamowicz SA, Titze IR, et al. Experimental approaches to vocal fold alteration: introduction to the minithyrotomy. Ann Otol Rhinol Laryngol. 1999;108:1–9.
14. Isshiki N, Ishikawa T. Diagnostic value of tomography in unilateral vocal cord paralysis. Laryngoscope. 1976;86:1573–8.
15. Bryant NJ, Gracco C, Sasaki CT, Vining E. MRI evaluation of vocal fold paralysis before and after type I thyroplasty. Laryngoscope. 1996;106:1386–92.
16. Laccourreye O, Bély N, Crevier-Buchman L, Brasnu D, Halimi P. Computerized tomography of the glottis after intracordal autologous fat injection. J Laryngol Otol. 1998;112:971–2.
17. Fang TJ, Lee LA, Wang CJ, Li HY, Chiang HC. Intracordal fat assessment by 3-dimensional imaging after autologous fat injection in patients with thyroidectomy-induced unilateral vocal cord paralysis. Surgery. 2009;146:82–7.
18. Safak MA, Gocmen H, Korkmaz H, Kilic R. Computerized tomographic alignment of silastic implant in type 1 thyroplasty. Am J Otolaryngol. 2000;21:179–83.
19. Yumoto E, Sanuki T, Hyodo M, Yasuhara Y, Ochi T. Three-dimensional endoscopic mode for observation of laryngeal structures by helical computed tomography. Laryngoscope. 1997;107:1530–7.
20. Yumoto E, Sanuki T, Hyodo M. Three-dimensional endoscopic images of vocal fold paralysis by computed tomography. Arch Otolaryngol Head Neck Surg. 1999;125:883–90.
21. Yumoto E, Nakano K, Oyamada Y. Relationship between 3D behavior of the unilaterally paralyzed larynx and aerodynamic vocal function. Acta Otolaryngol. 2003;123:274–8.
22. Yumot E, Oyamada Y, Nakano K, Nakayama Y, Yamashita Y. Three-dimensional characteristics of the larynx with immobile vocal fold. Arch Otolaryngol Head Neck Surg. 2004;130:967–74.
23. Oyamada Y, Yumoto E, Nakano K, Goto H. Asymmetry of the vocal folds in patients with vocal fold immobility. Arch Otolaryngol Head Neck Surg. 2005;131:399–406.
24. Yumoto E, Sanuki T, Minoda R, Kumai Y, Nishimoto K. Glottal configuration in unilaterally paralyzed larynx and vocal function. Acta Otolaryngol. 2013;133:187–93.
25. Yumoto E, Sanuki T, Minoda R, Kumai Y, Nishimoto K, Kodama N. Over-adduction of the unaffected vocal fold during phonation in the unilaterally paralyzed larynx. Acta Otolaryngol. 2014;134(7):744–52.
26. Yamada M, Hirano M. Recurrent laryngeal nerve paralysis. A 10-year review of 564 patients. Auris Nasus Larynx. 1983;10(Suppl):1–15.
27. Tanaka S, Chijiwa K, Hirano M. Study on over-adduction of unaffected vocal fold in unilateral recurrent laryngeal nerve paralysis. Larynx Jpn. 1993;5:135–41. in Japanese.
28. Sellars IE, Keen EN. The anatomy and movements of the cricoarytenoid joint. Laryngoscope. 1978;88:667–74.
29. Kasperbauer JL. A biomechanical study of the human cricoarytenoid joint. Laryngoscope. 1998;108:1704–11.
30. Gacek M, Gacek RR. Cricoarytenoid joint mobility after chronic vocal cord paralysis. Laryngoscope. 1996;106:1528–30.
31. Müller A, Paulsen FP. Impact of vocal cord paralysis on cricoarytenoid joint. Ann Otol Rhinol Laryngol. 2002;111:896–901.
32. Yin SS, Qiu WW, Stucker FJ. Major patterns of laryngeal electromyography and their clinical application. Laryngoscope. 1997;107:126–36.
33. Min YB, Finnegan EM, Hoffman HT, Luschei ES, McCulloch TM. A preliminary study of the prognostic role of electromyography in laryngeal paralysis. Otolaryngol Head Neck Surg. 1994;111:770–5.
34. Sittel C, Stennert E, Thumfart WF, Dapunt U, Eckel HE. Prognostic value of laryngeal electromyography in vocal fold paralysis. Arch Otolaryngol Head Neck Surg. 2001;127:155–60.

35. Halum SL, Patel N, Smith TL, Jaradeh S, Toohil RJ, Merati AL. Laryngeal electromyography for adult unilateral vocal fold immobility: a survey of the American Broncho-Esophagological Association. Ann Otol Rhinol Laryngol. 2005;114:425–8.
36. Xu W, Han D, Hou L, Zhang L, Zhao G. Value of laryngeal electromyography in diagnosis of vocal fold immobility. Ann Otol Rhinol Laryngol. 2007;116:576–81.
37. Wang CC, Chang MH, Wang CP, Liu SA. Prognostic indicators of unilateral vocal fold paralysis. Arch Otolaryngol Head Neck Surg. 2008;134:380–8.
38. Grosheva M, Wittekindt C, Potoschnig C, Lindenthaler W, Guntinas-Lichius O. Evaluation of peripheral vocal cord paralysis by electromyography. Laryngosscope. 2008;118:987–90.
39. Blitzer A, Crumley RL, Dailey SH, Ford CN, Floeter MK, Hillel AD, Hoffmann HT, et al. Recommendations of the Neurolaryngology Study Group on laryngeal electromyography. Otolaryngol Head Neck Surg. 2009;140:782–93.
40. Sanuki T, Yumoto E, Nishimoto K, Minoda R. Laryngeal muscle activity in unilateral vocal fold paralysis patients using electromyography and coronal reconstructed images. Otolaryngol Head Neck Surg. 2014;150:625–30.
41. Hirano M, Ohala J. Use of hooked-wire electrodes for electromyography of the intrinsic laryngeal muscles. J Speech Hear Res. 1969;12:362–73.
42. Munin MC, Rosen CA, Zullo T. Utility of laryngeal electromyography in predicting recovery after vocal fold paralysis. Arch Phys Med Rehabil. 2003;84:1150–3.
43. Smith LJ, Rosen CA, Niyonkuru C, Munin MC. Quantitative electromyography improves prediction in vocal fold paralysis. Laryngoscope. 2012;122.834–9.

Chapter 5
Surgical Treatment of Unilateral Vocal Fold Paralysis; Reinnervation of the Thyroarytenoid Muscle

Abstract The author sought to achieve laryngeal reinnervation, with or without arytenoid adduction (AA), to treat severe breathy dysphonia caused by unilateral vocal fold paralysis. One surgical approach is primary reconstruction of the recurrent laryngeal nerve (RLN) immediately after extirpation of a thyroid or other malignant tumor. The RLN is reconstructed via direct suturing, interpolation of a free nerve graft between the severed stumps of the RLN, or transfer of the ansa cervicalis nerve (ACN). Another strategy features delayed reinnervation of the larynx in combination with AA. Nerve–muscle pedicle flap implantation into the thyroarytenoid muscle (a technique refined by the author) will also be described. This technique and nerve transfer involving the ACN both deliver excellent vocal function several months postoperatively. Laryngeal edema after AA attains its maximum extent on postoperative day (POD) 3 and then gradually (and significantly) subsides to POD 7. Both AA and type I thyroplasty negatively affect respiratory functioning, although no patient experienced dyspneic symptoms when performing daily activities.

Keywords Laryngeal reinnervation • Thyroplastic surgery • Surgical technique • Laryngeal edema • Respiratory function

5.1 Introduction

Many surgical methods including type I thyroplasty, intracordal injection, arytenoid adduction (AA), and combinations thereof have been used to treat breathy hoarseness caused by unilateral vocal fold paralysis (UVFP). These methods aim to close the glottal gap and increase the thickness of the affected vocal fold. Chapter 1 identified several areas that are inadequately addressed by conventional phonosurgery, emphasizing the need to refine current surgical techniques. The thyroarytenoid (TA) muscle plays several important roles in adjusting the vertical thickness (the medial–inferior bulge) and in controlling the physical properties of the vocal fold. In

---

Electronic supplementary material The online version of this chapter (doi: 10.1007/978-4-431-55354-0_5) contains supplementary material, which is available to authorized users.

© Springer Japan 2015

E. Yumoto, *Pathophysiology and Surgical Treatment of Unilateral Vocal Fold Paralysis*, DOI 10.1007/978-4-431-55354-0_5

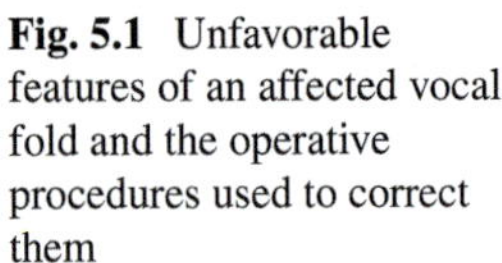
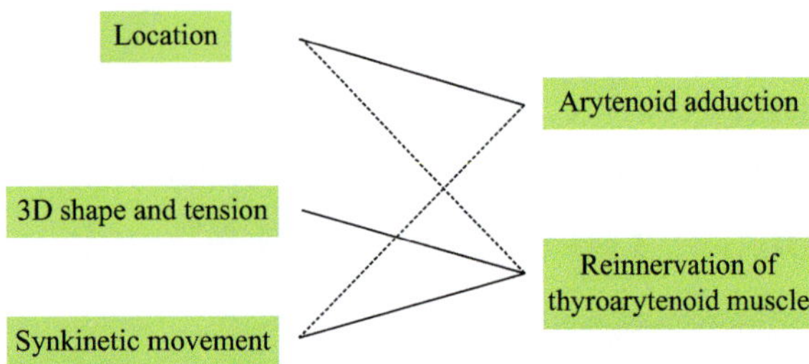

Fig. 5.1 Unfavorable features of an affected vocal fold and the operative procedures used to correct them

particular, the TA muscle regulates the cover tension and stiffness of the entire vocal fold. Thus, recovery of TA muscle contraction may be indispensable, in combination with median localization of the vocal fold, to restore a normal voice.

Figure 5.1 shows that AA rotates the affected vocal fold to the median position and prevents abduction of this fold secondary to type C synkinesis (abduction during phonation caused by misdirected nerve regeneration (see Chap. 4, Sect. 4.3.2)). Reinnervation of the TA muscle restores the medial–inferior bulge, adjusts the overall tension, and stabilizes the median location of the fold, because of reinforcement of the TA muscle contraction during phonation. This chapter will describe the author's experience regarding treatment of paralytic dysphonia, with the primary intent of recovery of normal voice. Reinnervation of the TA muscle, often combined with AA, was the mainstay of treatment. Perioperative complications and changes in respiratory functioning after phonosurgery will also be described.

5.2   The Basic Policy

Figure 5.2 is a flow chart outlining how the author selected an operative procedure for treatment of breathy dysphonia caused by UVFP. If a thyroid or other malignant neck tumor is to be extirpated, nerve reconstruction should be performed immediately after recurrent laryngeal nerve (RLN) resection. In such instances, the period from UVFP onset to RLN reconstruction is relatively short (often less than a few months), and excellent vocal outcomes may be expected, even in the absence of AA [1, 2]. In patients with persistent UVFP, nerve reconstruction is usually combined with AA for three principal reasons. The first reason is that facilitation of TA contraction during phonation, via reinnervation, affords a better voice than performance of AA alone or AA combined with medialization thyroplasty (intracordal injection or type I thyroplasty). The second reason is that combination therapy allows a patient to perceive voice improvement soon after surgery, although the voice is not normal at this time. This is important because the effects of reinnervation are not apparent for several months. The third reason is that even if reinnervation does not positively affect voice quality, conventional augmentation can still be undertaken.

When the ansa cervicalis nerve (ACN) and the sternohyoid (SH) muscle are both unavailable, conventional framework surgeries such as AA, with or without

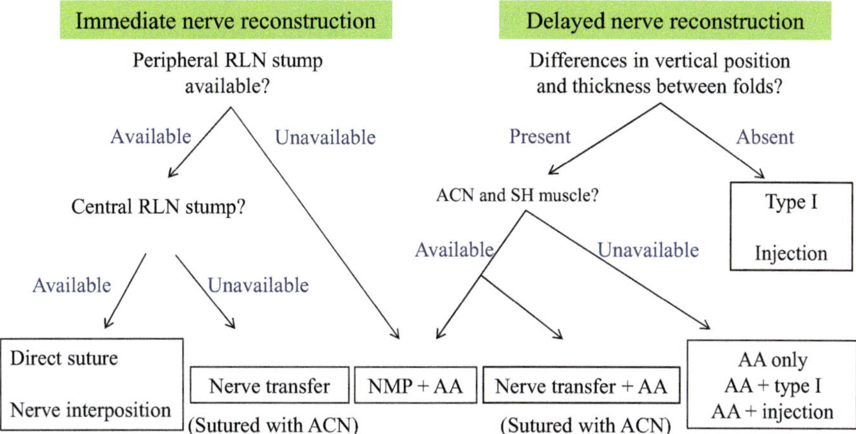

Fig. 5.2 Selection of an operative procedure to treat breathy dysphonia caused by unilateral vocal fold paralysis. *RLN* recurrent laryngeal nerve, *ACN* ansa cervicalis nerve, *NMP* nerve–muscle flap implantation, *AA* arytenoid adduction, *SH* sternohyoid, *Type I* type I thyroplasty, *Injection* intra-cordal injection

Fig. 5.3 Manual compression test

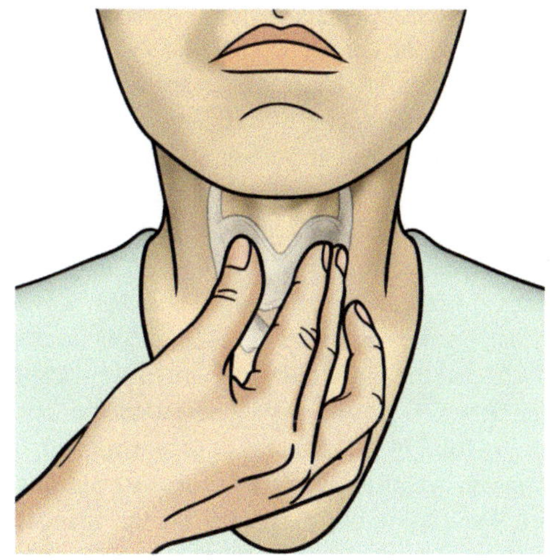

medialization thyroplasty, are performed. If the differences in the vertical positions and thicknesses of the two vocal folds are minimal during phonation, medialization laryngoplasty is indicated. Three-dimensional (3D) vocal fold configurations were assessed on the 3D computed tomographic images described in Chap. 4. If manual finger compression of the thyroid alae helps to improve the voice (Fig. 5.3) [3], the surgical outcome may well be favorable. In addition, this test helps the patient understand what the operation seeks to achieve.

5.3 Primary Reconstruction of the RLN

UVFP is often caused by invasion of the RLN by thyroid cancer or other malignant metastatic lesions of the neck. Furthermore, even if UVFP is not evident preoperatively, a tumor may be found, intraoperatively, to adhere firmly to the RLN, necessitating removal of the involved RLN region to ensure total cancer extirpation. The generally accepted management procedure for such patients who develop UVFP is the observation for several months after surgery; phonosurgical procedures are reserved for patients who desire voice improvement [4]. Breathy hoarseness improves after conventional phonosurgical treatments including intracordal injection, type I thyroplasty, AA, and combinations thereof, but voice quality does not attain a normal level, and long-term benefits cannot be guaranteed. Beginning in 1995, the author began to reconstruct severed RLNs immediately after extirpation of malignant lesions; the method is shown in Fig. 5.2.

5.3.1 Operative Procedures

The distal branch of the RLN is preserved to the maximal extent possible when a tumor invading the RLN is resected. When the nerve is transected at the entrance thereof to the larynx, the adductor branch of the RLN is identified by removing the inferior-posterior portion of the thyroid cartilage after disconnection of the cricothyroid joint. Because the adductor branch is thin, it is sometimes difficult to link the nerve stumps with three stitches. If both ends are appropriately fitted, one or two stitches may yield good postoperative vocal results. Direct suture of both stumps is technically and functionally possible only when the gap between the ends is less than 5 mm, because tension at the suture site is unacceptable. A free nerve graft is placed between the severed ends if direct anastomosis is not possible. A segment of the great auricular nerve (GAN) usually serves as such a graft (Fig. 5.4) because the graft surgical field is close to the RLN, and the GAN and RLN are of similar diameter. The third method is nerve transfer, in which the ACN is sutured to the peripheral end of the RLN when the other end of the RLN is unavailable for reconstruction. Nerve interposition is preferred to nerve transfer, because the motor supply to the intrinsic laryngeal muscles originates from the RLN and not the ACN. We believe that using the RLN as the regenerating nerve is better for restoring normal vocal function than other methods (including anastomosis with the ACN). In a few patients in whom the peripheral end of the RLN was unavailable for reconstruction, we performed nerve–muscle pedicle (NMP) flap implantation combined with AA. Figure 2.6 illustrates the methods used for laryngeal reinnervation.

The superior root of the ACN is located dorsal to the anterior belly of the omohyoid (OH) muscle and anterior to the internal jugular vein. The ACN is followed caudally until that nerve branch enters the sternohyoid (SH) muscle after looping around the inferior root (Fig. 5.5). A main branch is utilized for anastomosis with the peripheral end of the RLN. This step is performed under microscopic guidance to ensure an exact fit between the cut ends of the nerve fibers; between two and four ties of 9-0 nylon thread are placed.

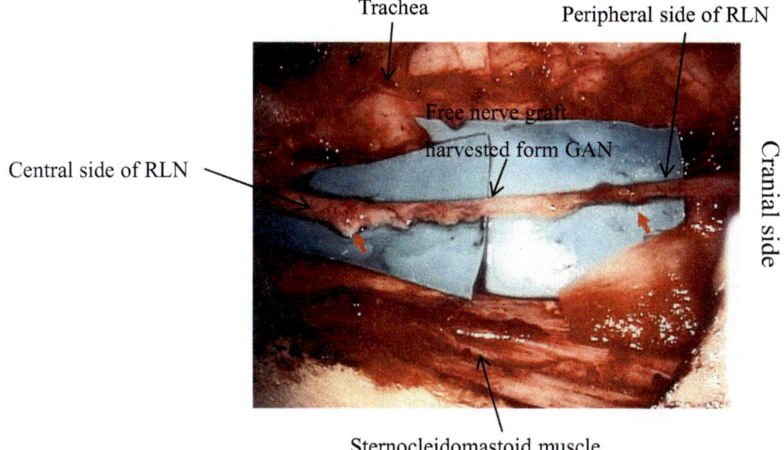

Fig. 5.4 Nerve interposition between the severed ends of the recurrent laryngeal nerve (RLN). A 39 year old female underwent total thyroidectomy together with RLN resection 3 months after onset of left vocal fold paralysis. The *red arrows* indicate the suturing sites. *GAN* great auricular nerve

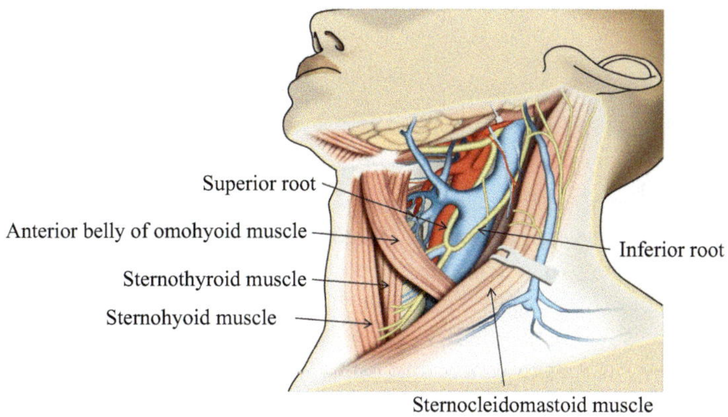

Fig. 5.5 Schematic drawing of the left ansa cervicalis nerve (ACN)

5.3.2   Subjects

Thirty-two patients underwent primary nerve reconstruction at the Department of Otolaryngology-Head and Neck Surgery, Kumamoto University Hospital, between March 2000 and March 2014. Table 5.1 shows the clinical profiles of these patients. In 19 patients, the duration of UVFP prior to surgery ranged from 1 to 62 months (median: 3.5 months); thus, most patients underwent nerve reconstruction within a few months after onset of UVFP. The ACN was utilized for nerve transfer in 17

Table 5.1 Demographic data of patients who underwent immediate recurrent laryngeal nerve reconstruction

Gender	9 males, 23 females
Age	18–86 years (60.4 ± 15.8)
Affected side	Left: 16, right: 16
Causes of vocal fold paralysis	Thyroid cancer: 25
	Metastatic cancer: 5
	(Esophageal cancer: 2, uterus/breast: 1 each)
	Vagus tumor: 2
	Mediastinal tumor: 1
Vocal fold paralysis before surgery	Present: 19 (7.9 ± 13.2, 3.5 months)[a]
	Absent: 12
	Unexplained: 1
Nerve reconstruction	Nerve transfer: 17
	Nerve interposition: 10
	Direct suture: 5

[a]Mean ± standard deviation and median value of duration of paralysis before surgery

patients, and in 1 patient with uterine cancer metastasis, the ACN of the unaffected side was moved to anastomose with the contralateral peripheral RLN stump.

5.3.3   Assessment of Vocal Function

The vocal function of each patient was assessed in terms of aerodynamics, acoustic analysis, and auditory impression, both before surgery and 1, 6, and 12 months postoperatively. The parameters measured were maximum phonation time (MPT), mean airflow rate (MFR), jitter, shimmer, harmonics-to-noise ratio (HNR), grade overall, greatness (using the GRBAS scale, which is an acronym for grade overall, rough, breathy, asthenic, and strained; 0 = normal, 1 = slight, 2 = moderate, 3 = extreme; see Sect. 4.2), and range of pitch. Auditory perceptual assessment using the GRBAS scale was conducted by three different listeners in random order. The mean values of G and B were recorded for each patient. Because the patients varied in terms of the presence or duration of UVFP prior to surgery, we examined vocal function after nerve reconstruction. The Mann–Whitney test was used for statistical analysis, and P < 0.05 was considered statistically significant. Table 5.2 shows the mean ranges of vocal function (except for jitter, shimmer, and HNR) of healthy Japanese men and women aged 50–59 years [5]. The normal ranges of acoustic parameters were taken from the manufacturer's practical guide to the Multi-Dimensional Voice Program (Kay-Pentax).

Temporal changes in the vocal functions of 22 patients, who underwent primary RLN reconstruction and who were followed-up over 12 months, are shown in Figs. 5.6, 5.7, 5.8, and 5.9. All vocal parameters exhibited continuous and significant improvement during the 12-month follow-up period. Although jitter and shimmer

Table 5.2 Normal ranges of vocal function

	Male	Female
MPT (second)	12.5–30.4	14.2–19.8
MFR (mL/s)	113–262	99–173
Pitch range (semitone)	18.2–28.6	18.7–30.4
Jitter	<1.04 %	
Shimmer	<3.81 %	
HNR	7.2 dB<	

MPT maximum phonation time, *MFR* mean airflow rate, *HNR* harmonics-to-noise ratio

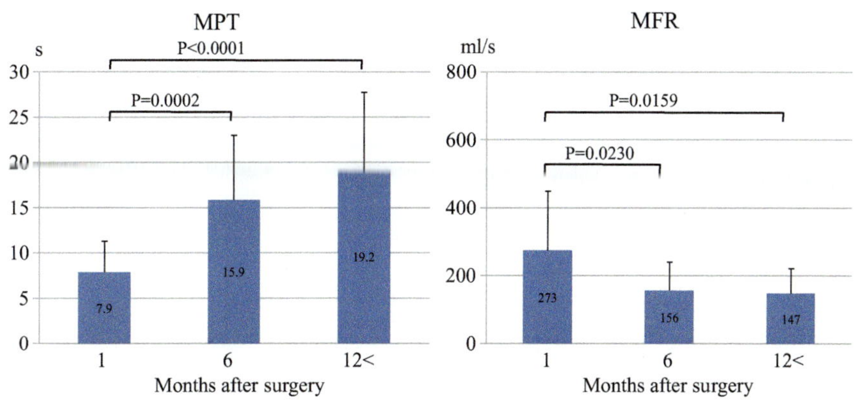

Fig. 5.6 Maximum phonation time (MPT) and mean airflow rate (MFR) of 22 patients who underwent primary reconstruction of the recurrent laryngeal nerve and were followed-up over 12 months. The *number* in each bar indicates the average and the *line above* the bar the standard deviation

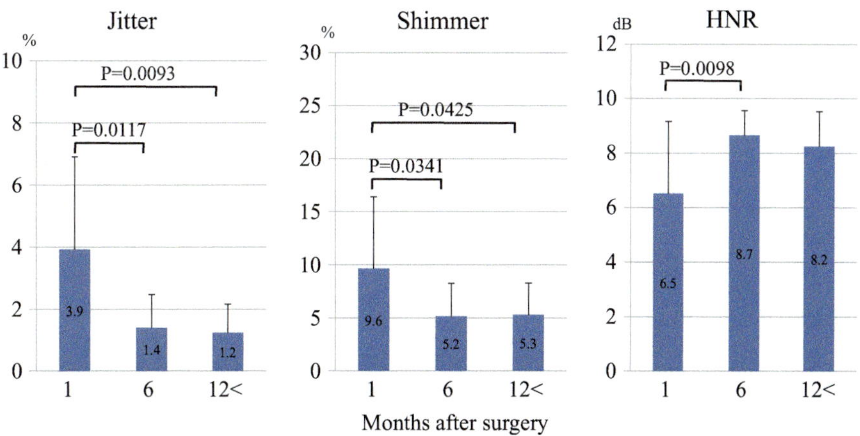

Fig. 5.7 Jitter, shimmer, and harmonics-to-noise ratio (HNR) of 22 patients who underwent primary reconstruction of the recurrent laryngeal nerve and were followed-up over 12 months. The *number* in each bar indicates the average and the *line above* the bar the standard deviation

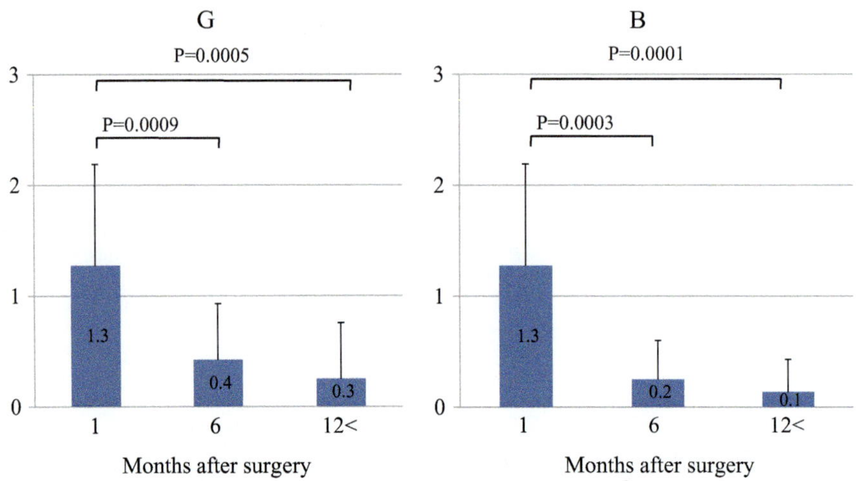

Fig. 5.8 G (grade overall) and B (breathiness) of 22 patients who underwent primary reconstruction of the recurrent laryngeal nerve and were followed-up over 12 months. The *number* in each bar indicates the average and the *line above* the bar the standard deviation

Fig. 5.9 The pitch range of 22 patients who underwent primary reconstruction of the recurrent laryngeal nerve and were followed-up over 12 months. The *number* in each bar indicates the average and the *line above* the bar the standard deviation

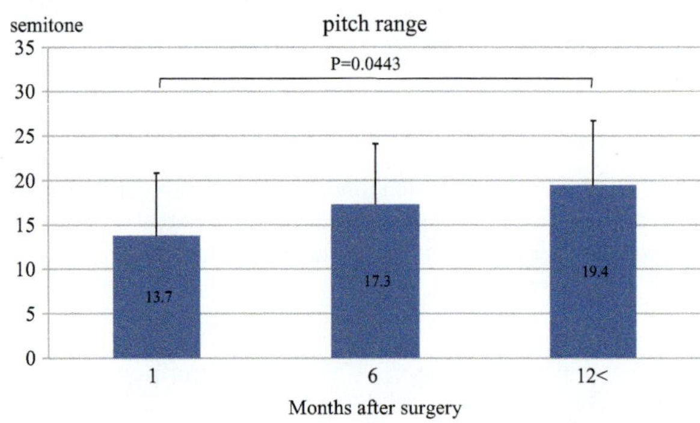

also significantly improved, the normal ranges of these parameters were not attained. However, all other parameters recovered to values within the normal ranges by 12 months after surgery.

5.3.4   Comments

Generally, the sooner a functional connection is made between a regenerating axon and a muscle fiber, the more likely it is that the extent of functional recovery of the muscle will be close to normal. Currently, however, no definitive clinical data are available on how long it is acceptable to wait from onset of UVFP to nerve reconstruction ensuring functional recovery of the muscle. The longest such interval in the present series was 14 months in a patient who had thyroid papillary cancer (thus delaying reinnervation); vocal function recovered to normal over the 12-month follow-up period. Of the nine patients in the report by Maronian et al. [6] who underwent laryngeal reinnervation procedures, eight developed a normal or improved voice. The interval between UVFP onset and surgery exceeded 12 months in all but one case. The longest interval was 9 years, after which the voice was noted to have improved. Denervation usually causes a drastic reduction in muscle fiber numbers and, ultimately, the total loss thereof. However, the duration of atrophy of human intrinsic laryngeal muscles remains unclear, because this varies among muscles [7]. Further work is required to determine the longest duration from UVFP onset to reinnervation that allows successful RLN reconstruction.

Another concern is the unfavorable effect of long-lasting nerve compression. Two such cases were encountered in our present series. In both patients, the RLNs were flat at the site of tumor adhesion because of chronic compression. One patient underwent nerve transfer using the intact ACN and experienced excellent vocal function postoperatively. The other patient underwent direct anastomosis of the severed ends because the gap was less than 5 mm; limited improvement in vocal function was noted (MPT: 7.1 s, G: 1.3, B: 1.0). Endoneurial tubes within a macroscopically distorted nerve may also be distorted, resulting in suppression of nerve regeneration per se or growth of sprouting fibers into the endoneurial tubes. Although we only have little evidence, we believe that any portion of a nerve that has been flattened by tumor compression should be removed and nerve reconstruction should be performed to optimize functional recovery.

5.4   Delayed Reinnervation of the TA Muscle After Onset of UVFP

Those patients who suffer from breathy dysphonia caused by UVFP are indicated for phonosurgical treatment. An operative procedure was selected using the flow chart in Fig. 5.2.

5.4.1   Indication

Unless the ACN has been resected during prior surgery, reinnervation of the TA muscle is attempted together with AA. If the ACN cannot be bilaterally located because of the presence of cicatricial tissue, or if electrical stimulation of the ACN does not elicit SH muscle contraction, AA alone is performed, and type I thyroplasty or intracordal injection is scheduled for a later date.

5.4.2   Operative Procedures for TA Muscle Reinnervation Combined with AA

5.4.2.1   Nerve–Muscle Pedicle Flap Implantation (Fig. 5.10) Combined with AA [8]

A NMP flap supplies the nerve fibers that regenerate through the ACN into the target muscle; such regenerating fibers make functional connections with postsynaptic acetylcholine receptors (AchRs) within individual muscle fibers. In the human TA muscle, neuromuscular junctions (NMJs) are concentrated in a band around the mid-belly of the muscle [9]. Therefore, an NMP flap is best placed around this region so that the distance that regenerating nerve fibers must travel to reach the AchRs is minimized, and the maximum number of functional connections to NMJs may be established. As indicated in Fig. 5.11, the mid-portion of the window in the thyroid ala that is used for NMP flap implantation corresponds to the mid-belly of the TA muscle. The RLN branch enters the TA muscle just posterior to the mid-portion of the window.

Anesthesia

General anesthesia with endotracheal intubation is induced. The patient lies in a supine position with a pillow under the shoulder. Generally, endotracheal tubes of inner diameters 6 and 7 mm are used for female and male patients, respectively. Employment of a relatively thin tube allows the vocal fold to adduct passively during the anteroinferior pull of the muscular process of the arytenoid cartilage.

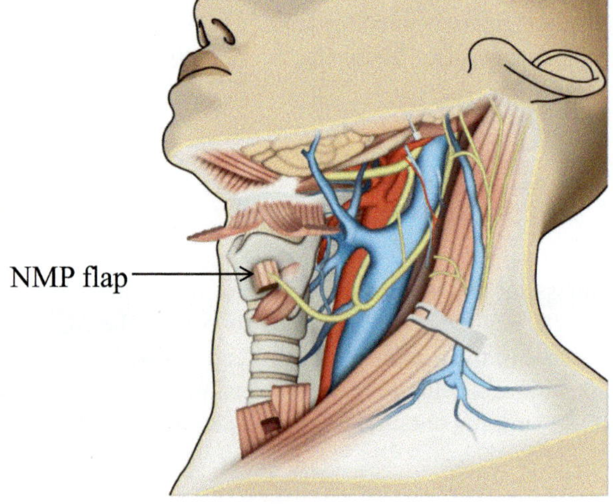

Fig. 5.10 Nerve–muscle pedicle (NMP) flap implantation. The flap is elevated cranially to attain the thyroid cartilage in a tension-free manner

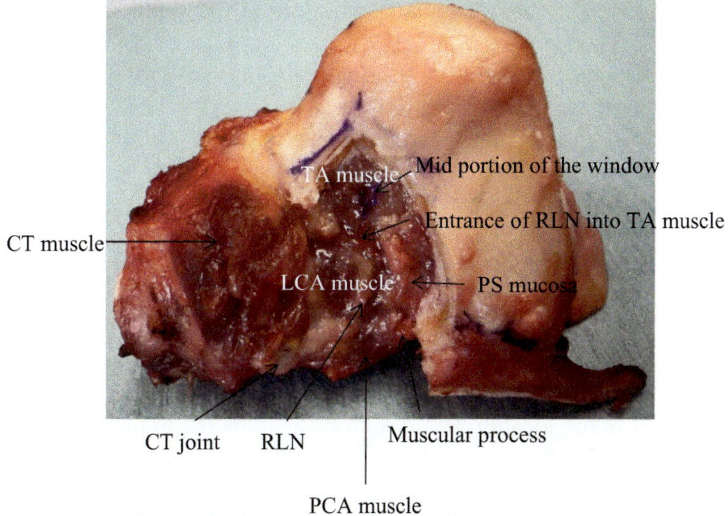

Fig. 5.11 Relationship between the mid-portion of a window in the thyroid ala used for NMP flap implantation and the thyroarytenoid muscle (the left side of the larynx, the right side was resected to treat laryngeal cancer in a 57-year-old male). The mid-portion of the window is marked with *blue pigment* (crystal violet). The lower part of the left thyroid ala was removed
CT cricothyroid, *LCA* lateral cricoarytenoid, *RLN* recurrent laryngeal nerve, *PS* pyriform sinus, *TA* thyroarytenoid

Skin Incision and Harvesting of the NMP Flap

An incision is made horizontally from the midline to the anterior margin of the sternocleidomastoid muscle at the level of the inferior one-fourth of the thyroid cartilage. The skin incision is approximately 5 cm long for females and 6 cm long for males. The sternocleidomastoid muscle is dissected anteriorly, exposing the internal jugular vein, where the ACN (the superior root) and the branch thereof to the omohyoid muscle are identified. The omohyoid muscle is transected, and the ACN is followed until the nerve enters the SH muscle. Electrical stimulation is applied to confirm the presence of nerve fibers innervating the SH muscle. A relatively thick AC branch to the SH muscle is harvested together with a 3×3 mm piece of the muscle at the point of the entrance of the nerve into the muscle; this is the NMP flap. The flap is elevated with meticulous care, and the course of the nerve reversed cranially to ensure that the flap attains the mid-portion of the thyroid ala without application of any tension. The inferior root of the ACN nerve is usually preserved.

Arytenoid Adduction

AA is performed using the method by Isshiki et al. [10] When approaching the muscular process, hydrocortisone sodium succinate (500 mg) is administered intravenously over 40–60 min to minimize postoperative mucosal edema. We do not open the cricoarytenoid joint. Care is taken to preserve the external branch of the superior laryngeal nerve and to avoid injury to the pyriform sinus mucosa. Opening of the paraglottic space and rotatory traction of the thyroid cartilage allow identification of the muscular process, via palpation along the posterior plate of the cricoid cartilage at a point approximately 1 cm cranially from the cricothyroid joint. Next, the muscular process is grasped with a pair of Adson forceps to confirm the passive mobility of the arytenoid. This step is necessary to estimate the degree of traction of the muscular process. Two 3-0 nylon threads are then placed through the muscular process and tied for later use.

Window Formation and Exposure of the TA Muscle Bundle

Figure 5.12 shows the location and design of the window in the thyroid ala. The window base is set 2–3 mm cranial to the lower edge of the thyroid ala. The medial edge is 5–7 mm distant from the midline, depending on the size of the thyroid ala, and the horizontal dimension of the window is 10 mm. The upper edge of the window is set 2 mm cranially from the estimated level of the vocal fold (Fig. 5.12, dotted line). The outer perichondrium is elevated and diamond-tip drills are used under

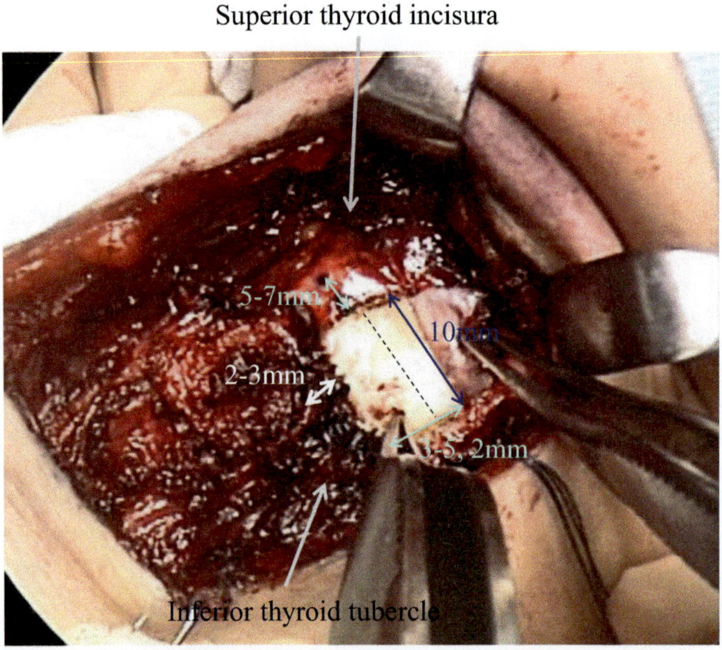

Fig. 5.12 Location and design of the window in the left thyroid ala. The dotted line indicates the estimated level of the vocal fold

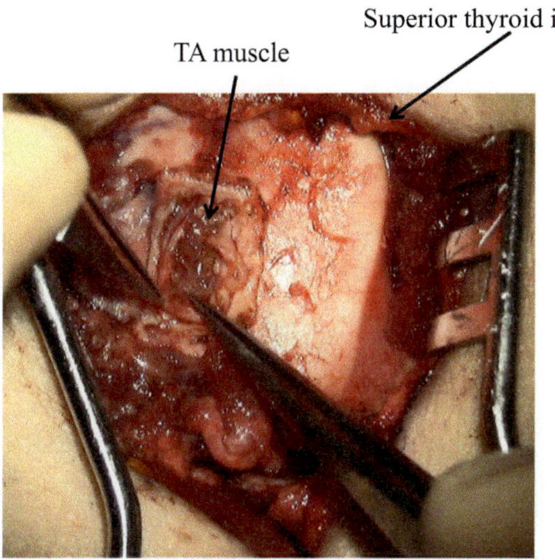

Fig. 5.13 Exposure of the thyroarytenoid (TA) muscle bundle through the window on the left side

microscopic guidance to create a window in which the inner perichondrium is intact. Next, that perichondrium is cut via electrocautery, with careful exposure of the TA muscle bundle to the maximal possible width, to establish sufficient contact between the NMP flap and the muscle (Fig. 5.13). A small pocket is created in the muscle at the point at which the NMP flap is sited.

Traction of the Muscular Process and NMP Flap Implantation

One of the nylon threads tied to the muscular process is introduced to the anterior surface of the thyroid ala, proceeding medially from the inferior tubercle. One end of the thread is passed through the lower edge of the window and the other is passed through the cricothyroid membrane. The second thread is likewise introduced, but in a slightly more medial position. The threads are used to pull the muscular process in a direction similar to that of the lateral cricoarytenoid (LCA) muscle, and are secured using a silicone shim.

The muscular region of the NMP flap is positioned in the window in a manner allowing the widest possible contact with the TA muscle and is secured to surrounding tissues using 8-0 nylon threads (Fig. 5.14, triangle). This step is crucial and is best performed under microscopic guidance. Subsequently, the window is covered with the outer perichondrium. Meticulous hemostasis is performed throughout the entire operation. A Penrose drain is placed in the wound; the drain is pointed toward the paraglottic space.

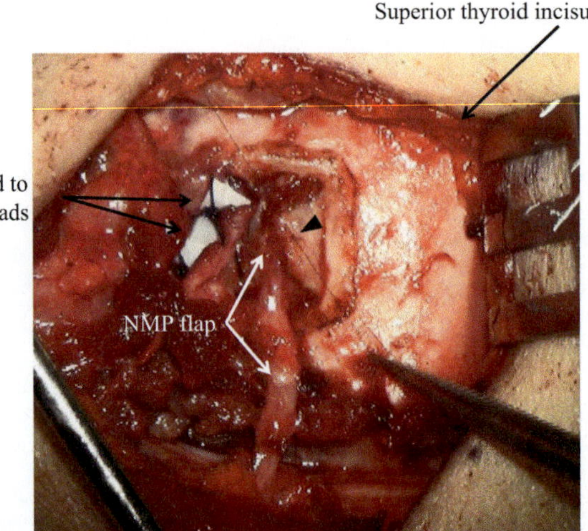

Fig. 5.14 Implantation of a nerve–muscle pedicle (NMP) flap on the left side. The triangle indicates an 8-0 nylon stitch between a piece of muscle and the inner perichondrium

5.4.2.2   Nerve Transfer Utilizing the ACN, Combined with AA [11]

General anesthesia with endotracheal intubation is induced. The overall procedure is similar to NMP flap implantation combined with AA, and below, only the differences between the two procedures will be discussed.

The skin incisions (5.5–6.0 cm and 6.5–7.0 cm in length for female and male patients, respectively) are slightly longer than those created during NMP flap implantation combined with AA. After the ACN is identified and elevated from the surrounding tissues, the RLN is isolated in the tracheoesophageal groove following elevation of the posterior border of the ipsilateral thyroid lobe. Meticulous hemostasis is important at this stage, because many blood vessels are located around the thyroid lobe. Two 3-0 nylon threads are tied through the muscular process, as described in the previous section. Particular attention is devoted to avoid injury to the pyriform sinus mucosa and the anterior division of the RLN at the surface of the posterior cricoid lamina (where the nerve is particularly vulnerable).

The proximal end of the ACN is anastomosed to the distal stump of the RLN with three or four stitches of 9-0 nylon thread, under a surgical microscope. Subsequently, traction is applied to pull the muscular process toward the anterior surface of the thyroid ala; two small adjacent holes are made in the thyroid ala. The posterior hole is placed just anterior to the inferior tubercle, and the anterior hole is placed 3 mm distant from the first hole. Nylon threads are introduced to the anterior surface of the thyroid ala through the two holes. One end of each thread is passed through a thyroid ala hole, and the other end is passed through the cricothyroid membrane. Next, the threads are tied over two small pieces of silicone to form two adjacent knots, after application of appropriate traction. Finally, two drains are placed in the wound, and the skin closed.

5.4.3   Subjects

Forty-three UVFP patients with severe breathy dysphonia underwent NMP flap implantation combined with AA between July 2002 and April 2011. In total, 10 patients were excluded from analysis: 2 required perioperative tracheostomy, 1 experienced wound opening caused by postoperative bleeding, 2 developed local infections after surgery, and 5 were lost to follow-up within 1 year. Consequently, 33 patients were finally enrolled (16 males, 17 females, age range 28–82 years, median age 59.5 ± 13.2 years). The average duration of UVFP prior to surgery was 24.9 months (range 1–366 months, median 9.0 months). The follow-up period ranged from 12 to 84 months (mean 29.0 months, median 26.0 months). The causes of UVFP are listed in Table 5.3.

Eleven UVFP patients with severe breathy dysphonia underwent nerve transfer combined with AA between October 2001 and November 2008. The primary etiologies of UVFP were associated with previous surgeries to treat a basal meningioma (1), esophageal cancer (1), a right vertebral artery aneurysm (1), a neck tumor (1), a vagal schwannoma (1), an aortic aneurysm (3), and a mediastinal tumor (1). The remaining two patients had left bulbar palsy (Wallenberg syndrome) (one) and an idiopathic etiology (one). Three patients were excluded from analysis; two patients experienced wound opening caused by postoperative bleeding, and one patient developed a recurrence of esophageal cancer. Thus, the vocal functions of eight patients (four males and four females) were followed-up over 2 years. The time from onset of paralysis to surgery ranged from 6 to 52 months (mean 23.0 ± 16.5 months).

Table 5.3 Causes of vocal fold paralysis

Causes of vocal fold paralysis	Number of patients	
Iatrogenic (postoperative)	27	
Thyroid cancer		9
Aortic aneurysm		7
Thymus tumor		2
Cerebral aneurysm		2
Esophageal cancer		2
Lung cancer		2
Graves disease		1
Mediastinal tumor		1
Vagal schwannoma		1
Subarachnoid hemorrhage	2	
Thyroid cancer	1	
Pulmonary tuberculosis	1	
Idiopathic	2	
Total	33	

5.4.4   *Assessment of Vocal Function*

The Mann–Whitney test was used in statistical analysis and P<0.05 was considered statistically significant.

5.4.4.1   NMP Flap Implantation Combined with AA

Of patients who underwent NMP flap implantation combined with AA, all postoperative voice parameters (measured at 1, 3, 6, 12, and 24 months) significantly improved compared to the preoperative data. Moreover, all parameters except MFR and pitch range exhibited significant improvement during the 2-year follow-up period (Figs. 5.15, 5.16, 5.17, and 5.18).

Two years after surgery, all MPT values were within the normal range and significantly improved compared to the values recorded 3 months postoperatively (Fig. 5.15). Jitter, shimmer, and HNR significantly improved during the follow-up period. The HNR values at 24 months were within the normal range, but jitter and shimmer were slightly above their normal ranges (Fig. 5.16). Auditory impressions (G and B) underwent continuous and significant improvement over time. In addition, such improvements persisted, as evidenced by comparing values measured at 3 months to those measured at 12 and 24 months and by comparing data collected at 6 months to those obtained at 24 months (Fig. 5.17).

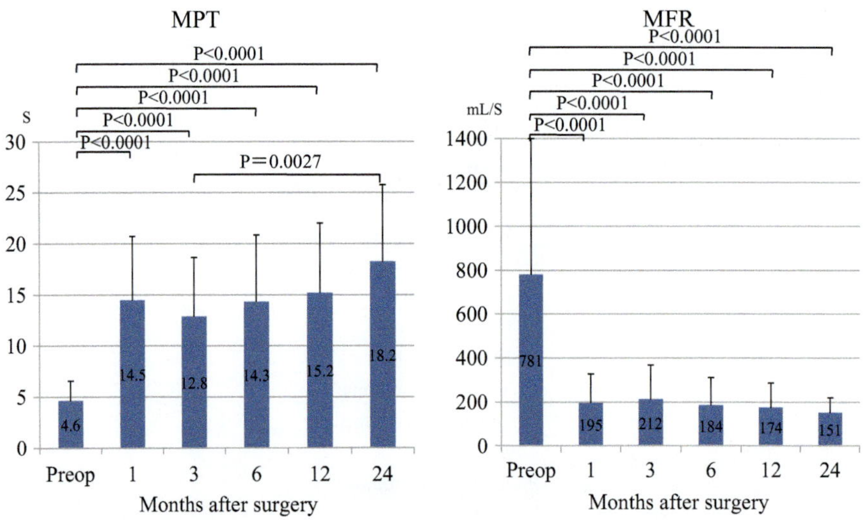

Fig. 5.15 Maximum phonation time (MPT) and mean airflow rate (MFR) of 33 patients who underwent nerve–muscle pedicle flap (NMP) implantation combined with arytenoid adduction. The *number* in each bar indicates the average and the *line above* the bar the standard deviation

Videos 5.1 and 5.2 are stroboscopic series of two representative cases who underwent NMP flap implantation combined with AA. The videos show the preoperative breathy dysphonia and recovery of voice over the follow-up period.

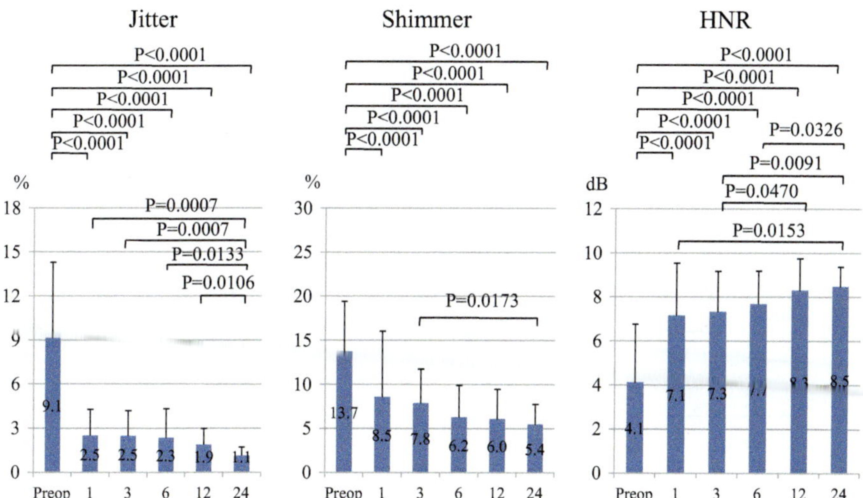

Fig. 5.16 Jitter, shimmer, and harmonics-to-noise ratio (HNR) of 33 patients who underwent nerve–muscle pedicle flap (NMP) implantation combined with arytenoid adduction. The *number* in each bar indicates the average and the *line above* the bar the standard deviation

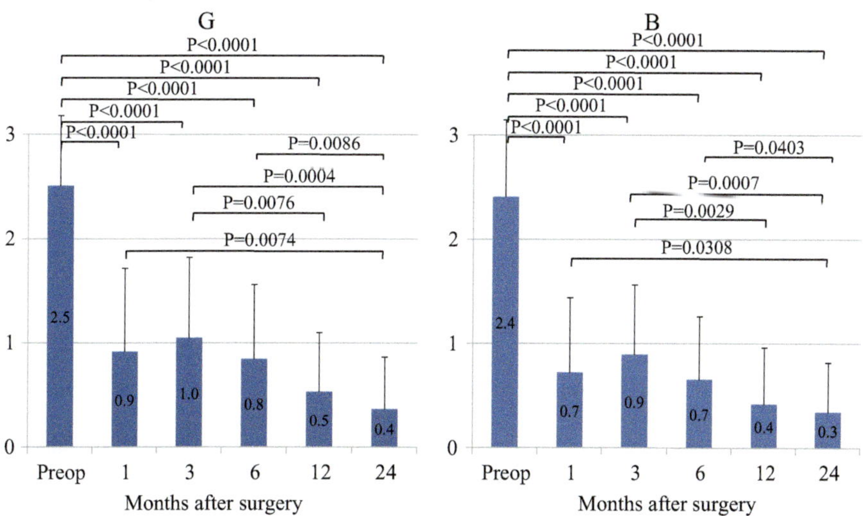

Fig. 5.17 G (grade overall) and B (breathiness) of 33 patients who underwent nerve--muscle pedicle flap (NMP) implantation combined with arytenoid adduction. The *number* in each bar indicates the average and the *line above* the bar the standard deviation

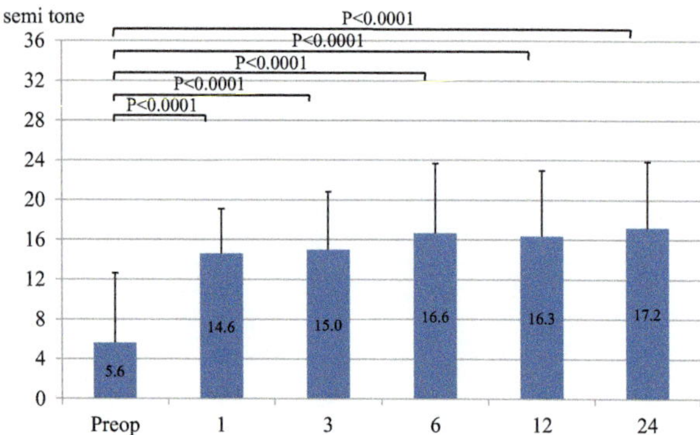

Fig. 5.18 Pitch range of 33 patients who underwent nerve–muscle pedicle flap (NMP) implantation combined with arytenoid adduction. The *number* in each bar indicates the average and the *line above* the bar the standard deviation

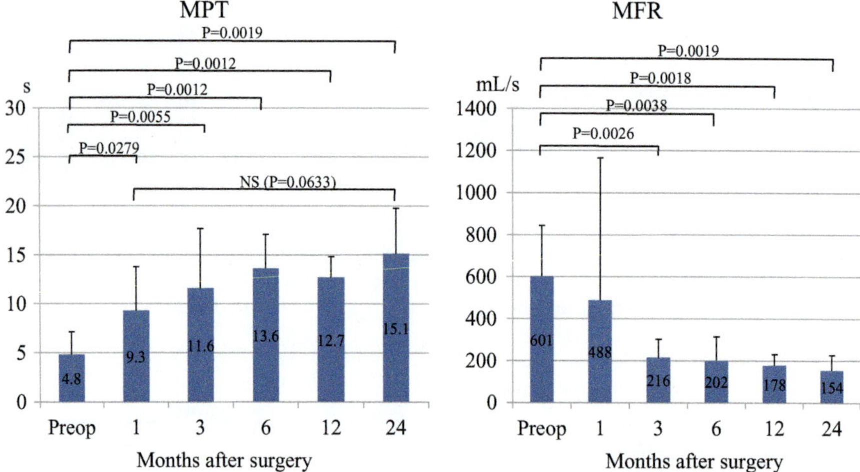

Fig. 5.19 Maximum phonation time (MPT) and mean airflow rate (MFR) of eight patients who underwent nerve transfer combined with arytenoid adduction. The *number* in each bar indicates the average and the *line above* the bar the standard deviation. *NS* not significant

5.4.4.2 Nerve Transfer Utilizing the ACN Combined with AA

Of the patients who underwent nerve transfer utilizing ACN combined with AA, all voice parameters except HNR significantly improved postoperatively. Shimmer and pitch range remained slightly outside their normal ranges, but all other parameters recovered to within the normal ranges. Acoustic parameters (jitter and shimmer), auditory impressions (G and B), and pitch range continued to significantly improve during the 2-year follow-up period (Figs. 5.19, 5.20, 5.21, and 5.22). Video 5.3 is a stroboscopic series of a case who underwent both ACN transfer and AA. The video shows the preoperative breathy dysphonia and recovery of a normal voice postoperatively.

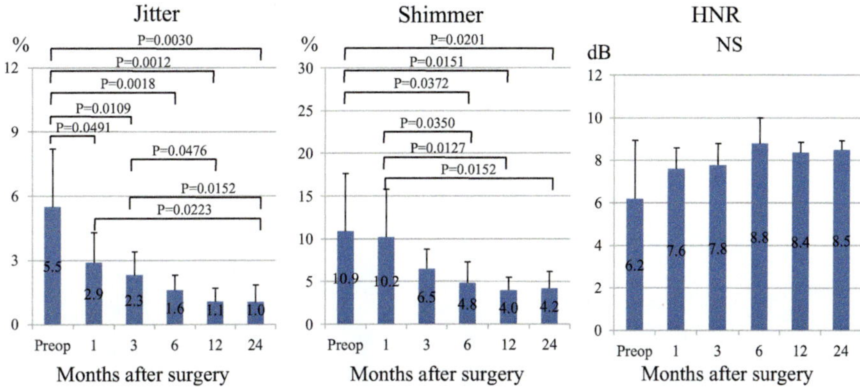

Fig. 5.20 Jitter, shimmer, and harmonics-to-noise ratio (HNR) of eight patients who underwent nerve transfer combined with arytenoid adduction. The *number* in each bar indicates the average and the *line above* the bar the standard deviation. *NS* not significant

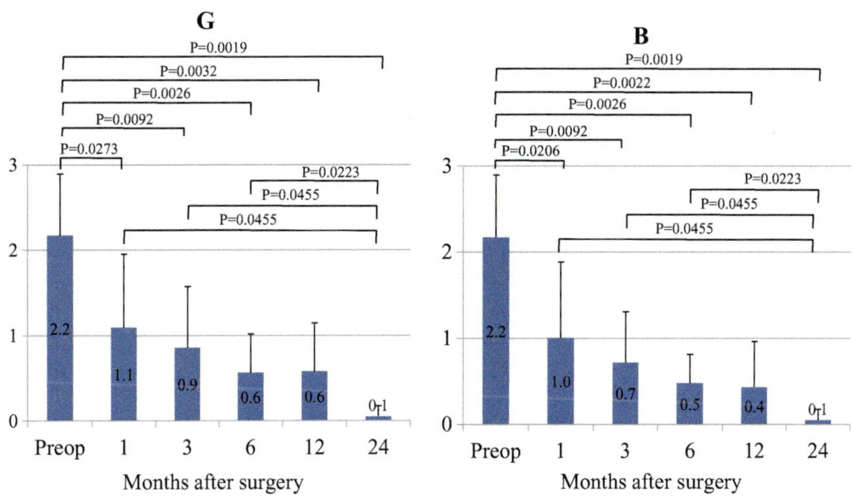

Fig. 5.21 G (grade overall) and B (breathiness) of eight patients who underwent nerve transfer combined with arytenoid adduction. The *number* in each bar indicates the average and the *line above* the bar the standard deviation

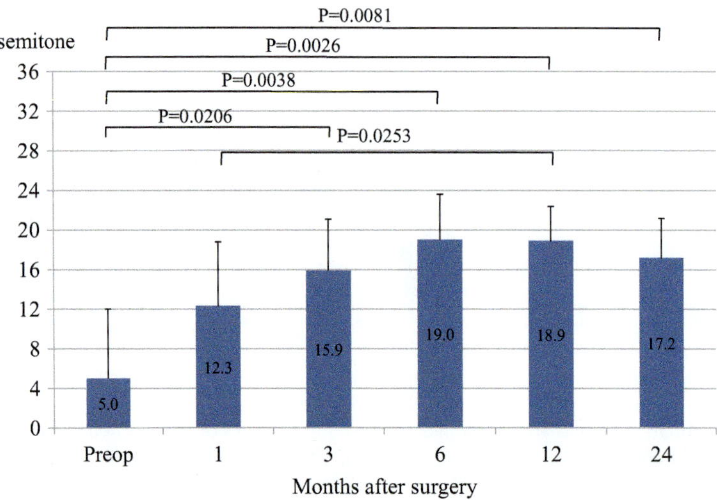

Fig. 5.22 Pitch range of eight patients who underwent nerve transfer combined with arytenoid adduction. The *number* in each bar indicates the average and the *line above* the bar the standard deviation

5.4.5 Comments

5.4.5.1 NMP Flap Implantation Combined with AA

Laryngeal reinnervation can increase the bulk and tension of the affected vocal fold, although the fold does not move. Of the various reinnervation procedures, the NMP method affords a practical method of reinnervation because the peripheral stump of the RLN is not required. However, as discussed in Chap. 2, Sect. 2.2.7.2, no surgeon has reported good vocal recovery after use of the NMP method (see the work of Tucker's group [12–16], May and Beery [17], and Maronian et al. [6]) Such data paucity may be associated with the lack of any consistent effect of the NMP method in animals. Some authors successfully used the NMP approach [18, 19], but others found it difficult to obtain reliable results [7, 20]. In a rat UVFP model, we found that the NMP method was effective when used to repair atrophic changes in the TA muscle, even in long-term denervated animals [21, 22]. Miyamaru et al. [22] also reported that stimulation of the ACN elicited TA muscle action potentials, which were attributed to successful reinnervation via the transferred ACN; the NMJs had been reconstructed. Formation and implantation of an NMP flap were carefully performed under microscopic guidance, and direct contact of the muscle flap with the TA muscle fibers was histologically confirmed. Based on such experimental results, we refined the NMP method and combined it with AA to treat UVFP.

Major differences are evident between our NMP method combined with AA and those of others [12–17]. First, we harvest an NMP flap from the SH muscle and the major ACN branch of that muscle; others use an NMP flap taken from the superior belly of the omohyoid muscle and the ACN branch thereof. [12–17] The lower portion of the SH muscle is invariably innervated by a prominent branch from the loop of the ACN. This branches further, and one major branch is both wider and contains more nerve fibers than the omohyoid branch [23]. Therefore, more regenerating axons may be expected to reach the target muscle. We always use electrical stimulation to confirm the presence of fibers innervating the SH muscle. Second, the TA muscle is the target muscle of both our technique and that of Tucker's group [14–16]. In contrast, May and Beery [17] sought to reinnervate the LCA muscle in an effort to medialize the affected vocal fold. In all, 7 of 29 patients in their series experienced no improvement. Third, all of the window opening, incision of the inner perichondrium, exposure of the TA muscle bundle, and fixation of the NMP flap are crucial steps and are performed with great care under microscopic guidance in our hands. Fourth, AA is performed together with NMP flap implantation to locate the affected vocal fold at the median position. To this end, Tucker [14–16] used type I thyroplasty, whereas May and Beery [17] did not combine flap implantation with any other surgery. All patients in our present series had relatively wide glottal gaps and thus required AA. Type I thyroplasty may not be indicated for combination with the NMP method, because successful reinnervation of the TA muscle already provides the desired increases in bulk and tension.

Further study focusing on electromyographic (EMG) examination is required to clarify the innervation status of the TA muscle. Currently, eight patients who underwent NMP flap implantation combined with AA have consented to EMG examinations after long-term follow-up. Table 5.4 shows patient profiles, EMG recruitment of the TA muscle during phonation, and pre- and post-operative vocal function. Recruitment was graded using the four-point scale of Munin et al. [24, 25], where 4+ indicates no recruitment, 3+ greatly decreased recruitment, 2+ moderately decreased recruitment, and 1+ mildly decreased activity with an interference pattern that is less than full. Three patients graded 4+ preoperatively exhibited 1+ recruitment 2 years after NMP placement; one rated 3+ preoperatively was graded 1+ after surgery, and two rated 2+ preoperatively improved to 1+. The other two patients, rated 2+ and 1+ preoperatively, exhibited the same extents of recruitment after surgery. Aerodynamic measurements and auditory evaluations (G and B) improved to near-normal levels in all patients. Figure 5.23 exemplifies recruitment in the TA muscle, from 4+ before surgery to 1+ 25 months postoperatively. More data from larger numbers of patients are required to confirm these preliminary results. In addition, long-term follow-up of vocal function, including aerodynamics, acoustic features, stroboscopic aspects, and patient self-evaluation, is underway in a larger number of patients.

5.4.5.2 Nerve Transfer Utilizing the ACN Combined with the AA

Chhetri et al. [26] compared AA+ACN-RLN anastomosis (10 patients) and AA alone (9 patients). Overall, no significant difference in any videostroboscopic parameter, aerodynamic measure, or perceptual rating was evident between the two

Table 5.4 Patients' profile who underwent nerve–muscle pedicle flap implantation combined with arytenoid adduction, electromyographic recruitment of thyroarytenoid muscle during phonation, and vocal function

No.	Age	Gender	Affected side	Causes of paralysis	Duration of paralysis (months)	Period from phonosurgery to EMG (months)	Recruitment	Aerodynamics		Auditory impression	
								MPT (s)	MFR (mL/s)	G	B
1	70	F	R	Post-op	14	Pre-op	4+	2.9	2,000	3.0	3.0
				Thyroid cancer		25	1+	18.2	94	0	0
2	51	F	R	Post-op	8	Pre-op	2+	6.3	223	1.7	1.7
				Subarachnoid hemorrhage		29	1+	12.0	238	0.0	0.0
3	48	M	L	Post-op	18	Pre-op	3+	3.5	731	2.0	2.0
				Thyroid cancer		27	1+	18.8	102	0	0
4	57	F	L	Post-op	60	Pre-op	1+	6.8	170	1.0	1.0
				Thyroid cancer		28	1+	14.5	214	0	0
5	71	M	L	Post-op	12	Pre-op	4+	3.0	2,000	3.0	3.0
				Aortic aneurysm		25	1+	11	158	0.3	0.3
6	37	F	L	Post-op	22	Pre-op	4+	6.3	398	2.0	2.0
				Grave's disease		24	1+	13.3	141	0.3	0.3
7	58	M	L	Post-op	8	Pre-op	2+	4.8	480	2.0	2.0
				Thyroid cancer		28	1+	14.8	233	0	0
8	66	F	L	Post-op	14	Pre-op	2+	2.8	420	3.0	3.0
				Thyroid cancer		33	2+	29.2	109	0	0

F female, *M* male, *R* right, *L* left, *MPT* maximum phonation time, *MFR* mean airflow rate, *G* grade overall, *B* breathiness
4+, absent recruitment; 3+, greatly decreased recruitment; 2+, moderately decreased recruitment; 1+, mildly decreased activity with a less than full interference pattern; 0, normal recruitment

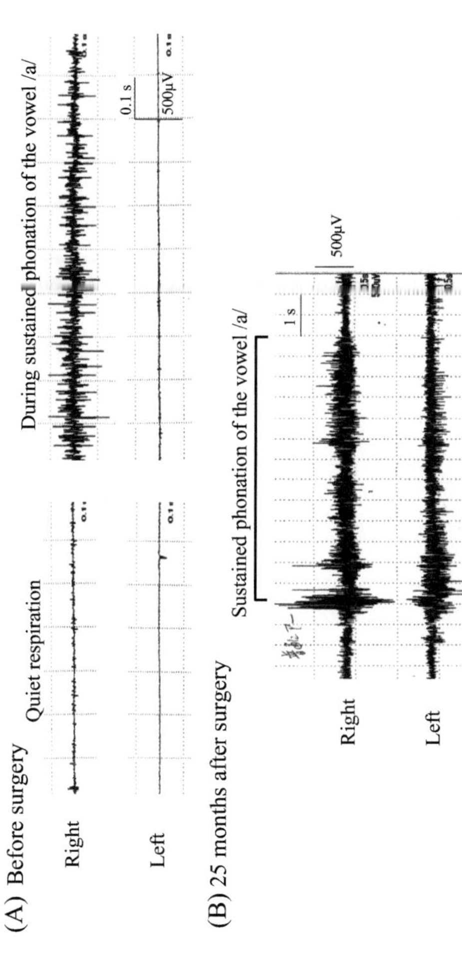

Fig. 5.23 Electromyographic activities of the thyroarytenoid muscle before and 25 months after NMP flap implantation and AA in a 71-year-old male with severe breathy dysphonia caused by left vocal fold paralysis (Patient 5 of Table 5.4)

groups. Although the cited authors speculated that this was attributable to the small number of patients treated, the most probable reason is likely to be variability of the follow-up period, which ranged from 3 to 36 months. In the combined group, 4 of 10 patients were examined within 8 months. Voice usually begins to improve 4–6 months after reinnervation [27] and is expected to further improve over at least 1 year postoperatively. Therefore, the cited report lacked adequate follow-up. Lorenz et al. [28] followed-up only 21 of 46 patients who underwent AA+ACN-RLN and reported significant improvements in vocal function 6, 12, and 18 months after surgery. However, detailed data were not provided. When we combine nerve transfer with AA, we note continuous and significant voice improvement over a 2-year follow-up period.

5.5 Complications After Surgery

5.5.1 Retrospective Review of Our Experience

Table 5.5 shows the number of patients who underwent framework surgeries (type I thyroplasty, AA, AA combined with type I thyroplasty, nerve transfer, NMP flap implantation); the number of operations performed; and the number of each type of complication that developed after application of each of the five modes of operation from March 1999 to August 2014.

No complication developed after 32 type I thyroplasties. Thus, all complications occurred after the use of AA or AA combined with another method. Hematomas formed in six patients, three of whom developed laryngeal edema and underwent tracheostomy with hematoma removal and hemostasis. Tracheostomy was not necessary in the other three patients, because early detection and prompt management of postoperative bleeding prevented development of laryngeal edema. Laceration of the pyriform sinus mucosa created salivary fistulae in two patients. One patient had undergone AA immediately after resection of invasive thyroid cancer and underwent mucosal closure operation 3 days later. The other patient only required conservative treatment, with local compressive dressing.

Overall, tracheostomy was required in nine patients. Three patients developed laryngeal edema after hematoma formation, as mentioned above. Two patients developed laryngeal edema 1 and 3 days after surgery, respectively, without hematoma formation. Such results made us decide to assess the day-to-day progression of laryngeal edema after AA; our results will be described in the next section (Sect. 5.5.2).

Limited abduction of the unoperated vocal fold was the cause of stridor in one patient. Thus, meticulous evaluation of the movements of both vocal folds is critically important. The cause of stridor in the remaining three patients was considered to be a laryngeal closure reflex triggered by esophageal regurgitation. Two of the three patients had previously undergone esophagectomy with gastric tube reconstruction and experienced sudden inspiratory distress, when eating 1 and 2 days after performance of AA and type I thyroplasty. The day after emergent tracheostomy,

Table 5.5 Number of patients with postoperative complication for each operation mode

Operation mode	Number of patients	Number of operations performed	Complication				
			Hematoma	Fistula	Stridor	Infection	Extrusion of implant
Type I	29[a]	32	0	0	0	0	0
AA	27	28	1	1[c]	2[b]	0	0
AA and type I	17	17	3[d]	0	3[e]	0	0
AA and nerve transfer	13	13	1	0	1	0	0
AA and NMP	92	92	1	1	3[f]	1	0
Total	149	182	6	2	9	0	0

Type I type I thyroplasty, *AA* arytenoid adduction, *NMP* nerve–muscle pedicle flap implantation, *Fistula* fistula of the pyriform sinus mucosa, *Stridor* tracheostomy was performed due to laryngeal edema

[a]10 patients underwent type I after AA was performed.

[b]One had hemorrhage and the other showed limited abductory movement of the unaffected vocal fold

[c]AA was performed immediately after removal of extensive thyroid cancer.

[d]One of them underwent tracheostomy.

[e]Glottal closure reflex or paradoxical vocal fold movement due to gastroesophageal reflux was the cause of dyspnea in 2 patients.

[f]Causes of stridor was paradoxical vocal fold movement due to gastroesophageal reflux, hematoma, and late-onset laryngeal edema.

both had adequately wide glottis, as revealed by laryngeal endoscopy. Videofluorography revealed strictures at the junctions between the duodenum and the gastric tube, with barium pooling above the strictures. Barium regurgitation was also noted. Based on these clinical courses and findings, a laryngeal closure reflex triggered by esophageal regurgitation is considered to be the most likely cause of the dyspneic attacks [29]. The UVFP of the third patient was caused by a post-subarachnoid hemorrhage operation; this patient developed sudden dyspnea several hours after AA and NMP flap implantation. The vocal fold on the healthy side was fixed at the median position, and a tracheostomy was performed. However, endoscopy performed on the following day revealed that the vocal fold on the healthy side was mobile and that the glottis was sufficiently wide to allow respiration. The cause of sudden dyspnea was inferred to be a laryngeal closure reflex triggered by esophageal regurgitation.

AA applied in combination with type I thyroplasty induced an element of laryngeal obstruction. Perie et al. [30] found that readjustment was required for production of a more natural voice and to maintain breath control, which may temporarily become destabilized. The cited authors suggested that changes in the position and thickness of the immobile vocal fold after thyroplastic surgery caused temporary disarrangements of laryngeal functions in the context of airway activity, swallowing, and phonation. Thus, we incorporated videofluorography into the test battery administered prior to AA in our hospital. If barium pooling is evident in the lower region of the esophagus, or if esophageal regurgitation is identified, mini-tracheostomy is recommended, especially in patients with histories of operations to treat esophageal cancer and those experiencing swallowing difficulties.

Table 5.6 summarizes the reported incidences of complications developing after type I thyroplasty and AA [31–37]. Extrusion of implant material occurred in 6–10 % of patients after type I thyroplasty. Severe stridor, triggering a need for tracheostomy, occurred in 2–6 % of patients after AA. Nito et al. [37] found that 51 (27.2 %) of 184 AA patients experienced varying degrees of dyspnea after surgery, although only 3 (1.6 %) required tracheostomy.

Table 5.6 Reported incidence of complication after type I thyroplasty (type I) and arytenoid adduction (AA)

Author	Year	Operation mode	Severe stridor due to laryngeal edema	Extrusion of implant
Tucker [31]	1993	Type I	6/60 (10.0 %)	4/60 (6.7 %)
Cotter [32]	1995	Type I	0	5/51 (9.8 %)
Abraham [33]	2001	Type I	0	7/98 (7.1 %)
Lin [34]	2009	Type I	1/17 (5.9 %)	–
Rosen [35]	1998	AA	57/1977 (2.9 %)	–
Weinman [35]	2000	AA	5/143 (3.5 %)	–
Abraham [33]	2001	AA+type I	4/96 (4.2 %)	–
Nito [37]	2008	AA	3/184 (1.6 %)	–

5.5.2   *Prospective Evaluation of Laryngeal Edema After AA [38]*

Unlike type I thyroplasty, AA involves dissection extending to the posterolateral larynx to allow access to the muscular process of the arytenoid cartilage. This, coupled with a permanently adducted vocal fold, may cause edema that compromises an already narrowed airway. In this section, the characteristics of the postoperative laryngeal airway are assessed by evaluating edema in three principal areas within the larynx, namely, the membranous vocal fold (MVF), the arytenoid mound (AM), and the pyriform sinus (PS) on the operated side. We developed a new videolaryngoscopic classification scheme to present our results. Figure 5.24 shows the four-point scale used to assess the extent of edema in the MVF, AM, and PS with 0 indicating none, 1 indicating mild, 2 indicating moderate, and 3 indicating severe. Scores 1–3 at each site are defined as follows:

MVF: 1 for confined edema (no contact with the opposite vocal fold), 2 for expanding edema (contact with less than one-half of the opposite vocal fold), and 3 for expanding edema (contact with more than one-half of the opposite vocal fold).

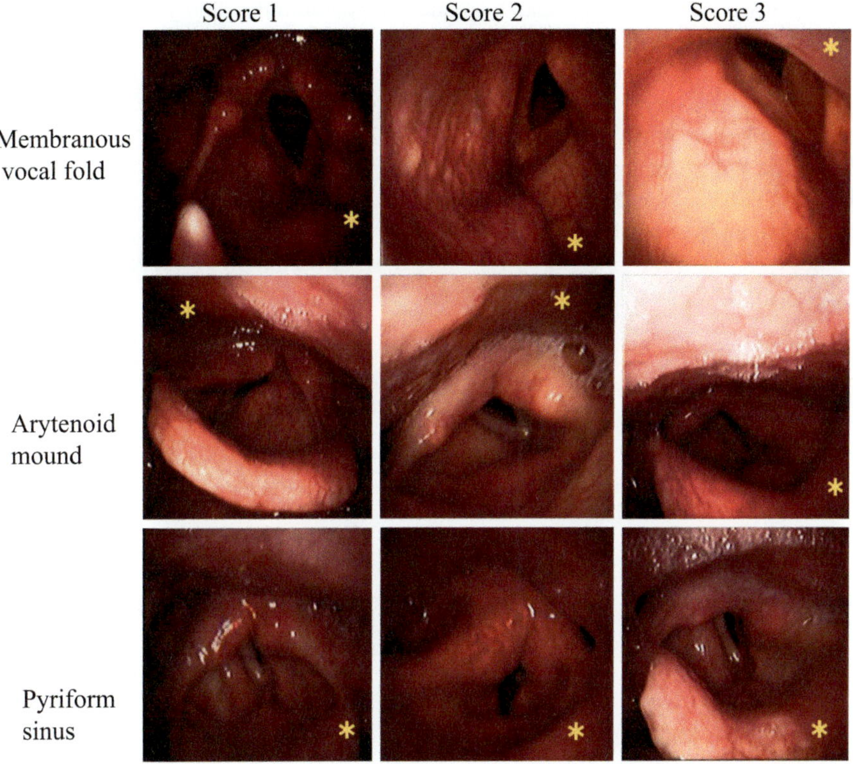

Fig. 5.24 Videolaryngoscopic scoring of the extent of edema in each of three laryngeal sites: the membranous vocal fold, the arytenoid mound, and the pyriform sinus. '*' indicates the operated side (Citation: Ref. [38])

AM: 1 for confined edema (of only the affected arytenoid mound), 2 for expanding edema (extending to the aryepiglottic fold), and 3 for expanding edema (extending to the aryepiglottic fold and base of the epiglottis).

PS: 1 for a visible PS space (but more shallow than that of the unaffected side), 2 for some visible space (the edematous mucosa obliterates more than one-half of the PS), and 3 for no visible space (the edematous mucosa completely obliterates the PS).

Nineteen consecutive UVFP patients who underwent AA alone (Group I: 6 patients) or in combination with reinnervation procedures (Group II: 3 treated via AA+nerve transfer and 10 via AA+NMP flap implantation) between February 2008 and August 2010, at Kumamoto University Hospital, were included. Postoperative laryngeal findings were recorded daily from postoperative day (POD) 1 for 10 days. Patients were observed during quiet breathing. The scope tip was placed over and at the level of the epiglottic laryngeal surface to view the AM and PS.

No postoperative complication, such as hematoma or wound infection, was encountered during hospitalization. No episode of airway obstruction requiring tracheostomy occurred. Postoperative edema was scored individually by three trained otolaryngologists in a blinded fashion and the final edema scores were the means of these three scores. A trend emerged over the 10-day postoperative period; edema was progressive at all three sites, attaining the highest level on POD 3 and then declining significantly from POD 3 to POD 7, as shown in Figs. 5.25, 5.26, and 5.27. The Wilcoxon signed rank test revealed that changes in the degree of edema between PODs 1–3 and PODs 3–7 were significant at all sites. The maximum degree of edema tended to be higher at all three sites in Group II with the following mean values (± SDs): MVF 2.43±0.42 vs. 2.33±0.61; AM 2.56±0.42 vs. 2.27±0.55; PS

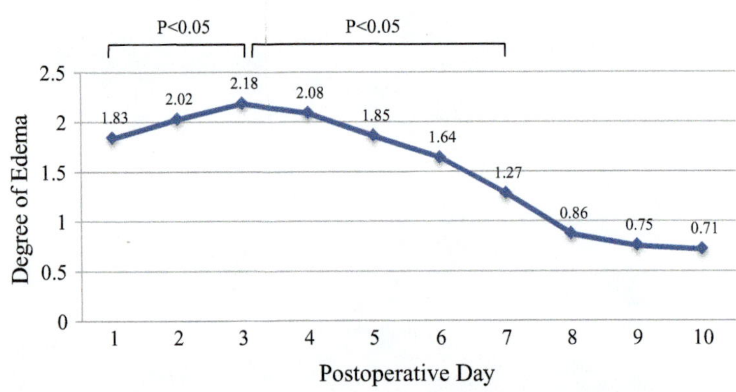

Fig. 5.25 Changes in the degree of membranous vocal fold edema (Citation: Ref. [38])

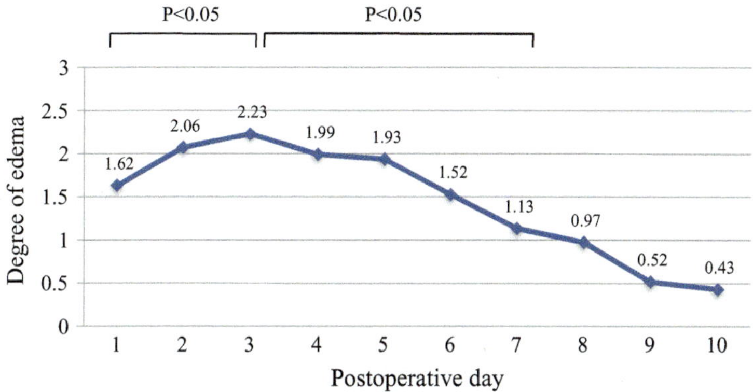

Fig. 5.26 Changes in the degree of arytenoid mound edema (Citation: Ref. [38])

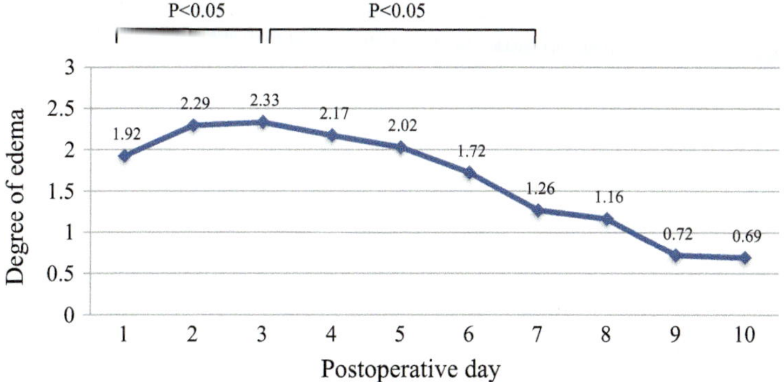

Fig. 5.27 Changes in the degree of pyriform sinus edema (Citation: Ref. [38])

2.63 ± 0.46 vs. 2.37 ± 0.51. The maximum edema time (the period of the day during which edema was elevated over the 10-day postoperative period, determined as the mean score of the three ratings) tended to be prolonged in Group II patients: MVF 3.27 ± 0.75 vs. 2.7 ± 1; AM 3.54 ± 0.78 vs. 2.4 ± 0.58; PS 3.27 ± 1.3 vs. 2.58 ± 0.97. However, the Mann–Whitney U test revealed no significant difference between the two groups.

Thus, we found that postoperative edema had a slow onset. Edema at all three studied sites is progressive, being maximal on POD 3, but usually did not trigger a need for airway intervention and gradually subsided through POD 10. However, considering the relatively late development of laryngeal edema (POD 3), it is recommended that patients be informed that swelling may continue to develop after the procedure. Should any respiratory difficulty be encountered within a week, patients should be encouraged to visit their clinicians or the nearest hospital for repeat scoping and work-up if needed.

5.6   Respiratory Function After Surgery

The aims of phonosurgeries including type I thyroplasty, AA, a combination of these approaches, and AA with reinnervation are augmentation and median fixation of the immobile vocal fold. Thus, the glottal aperture during inspiration after the immediate postoperative edema has subsided to be (in theory) smaller than that before surgery. However, inspiratory distress occurs only rarely and may manifest as esophageal regurgitation [29]. Nevertheless, the relatively narrow glottal aperture may influence the respiratory functioning of UVFP patients after phonosurgery. Respiratory functions were reported to be slightly deranged after intracordal injection and type I thyroplasty, but no apparent effect on patient activities was evident [30, 39–43]. No report on the effect of AA, either alone or combined with other methods, on respiratory function has appeared. In this section, the effects of thyroplastic surgeries, including type I thyroplasty and AA on respiratory functions, will be examined. The number of subjects studied to date is greater than that examined earlier [44].

Between March 1999 and December 2009, 87 patients underwent thyroplastic surgery to treat breathy dysphonia caused by UVFP at Kumamoto University Hospital. The thyroplastic surgical methods employed included type I thyroplasty, AA alone, a combination of AA with type I thyroplasty, and AA with NMP flap implantation [8]. Seventy-five patients who underwent respiratory function testing pre- and post-operatively were included in analysis. Table 5.7 summarizes the patient ages, genders, and the injured parts of the RLN, in terms of each type of surgery.

Respiratory functional testing was performed within 2 weeks prior to surgery and more than 6 weeks after surgery, thus when the postoperative local edema had subsided. The indices used in analysis included the ratio of forced expiratory volume in 1 s (FEV_1) to forced expiratory volume (FEV) (i.e., the $FEV_{1\%}$), peak expiratory flow rate (PEFR), and FEV_1/PEFR expressed as mL/L/min. The FEV_1/PEFR is <10 in normal subjects and >10 in patients with upper airway obstruction

Table 5.7 Age (mean ± SD) and the number of patients by gender and injured part of the recurrent laryngeal nerve for each type of surgery performed

Type of surgery	Number of patients	Age (years)	Gender		Injured part of RLN			
			Male	Female	Head	Neck	Thorax	Unknown
Type 1	7	66.6 ± 14.2	5	2	0	2	3	2
AA	14	61.1 ± 16.6	9	5	1	9	3	1
AA with Type I	14	58.9 ± 14.6	11	3	1	4	5	4
AA with NMP	40	59.0 ± 14.8	21	19	5	14	17	4

[45, 46]. $FEV_{1\%}$ and PEFR were expressed as ratios to the expected values based on gender, age, and height. Flow-volume loop examination during inspiration is not performed in the Pulmonary Center of Kumamoto University Hospital, because the results obtained during inhalation are much more variable than those obtained during expiration. When an upper airway obstruction is present, a large reduction in expiratory flow is only evident at a high lung volume; the PEFR becomes smaller, but the FEV_1 remains almost unchanged. Thus, any reduction in the PEFR would be greater than the reduction in FEV_1. This contrasts with what is found in patients with lower airway obstructions (such as asthma), in which the reductions in FEV_1 and PEFR are roughly proportional. Therefore, an increase in the $FEV_1/$PEFR index is to be expected when an upper airway obstruction is present. The paired Student's t-test was used for statistical comparisons of pre- and postoperative measurements.

Table 5.8 shows the means and standard deviations of the pre- and postoperative levels of $FEV_{1\%}$, PEFR, and $FEV_1/$PEFR in the four groups. In all groups, the $FEV_{1\%}$ and PEFR levels exhibited relatively small decreases postoperatively. Only four of the differences between pre- and postoperative values were significant: $FEV_{1\%}$ in the AA with type I thyroplasty group and PEFR in the three groups of type I thyroplasty, AA alone, and AA with NMP. The $FEV_1/$PEFR was less than 10 both pre- and postoperatively in all four groups, and the difference between the pre- and postoperative values was only significant in the AA with NMP group. Although no significant change in $FEV_{1\%}$ or $FEV_1/$PEFR was found, type I thyroplasty negatively affected postoperative respiratory function because the PEFR significantly decreased after that procedure.

The posterior glottis accounts for 50–60 % of the entire glottal area [47]. As AA moves the immobile vocal fold to the midline by rotating the arytenoid cartilage, the effect of AA on the glottis during inhalation may be greater than that of type I thyroplasty alone, which narrows the anterior glottis by pressing the membranous part of the vocal fold medially. One-way ANOVA did not reveal any significant difference in $FEV_{1\%}$, PEFR, or $FEV_1/$PEFR among the three groups in whom AA alone, AA with type I thyroplasty, or AA with NMP was performed. Therefore, all 68 patients were combined for statistical analysis. As shown in Table 5.9, the differences between pre- and postoperative measurements were significant for PEFR and $FEV_1/$PEFR. However, no patient complained of dyspneic symptoms when performing normal daily activities after surgery.

We have shown in this section that subclinical extrathoracic airway compromise may develop after thyroplastic surgery, although no patient reported dyspneic symptoms. Care should be taken when AA (with or without another vocal fold augmentation procedure) is planned for patients who intend to engage in strenuous physical activity.

Table 5.8 Means and standard deviations of pre- and postoperative measurements of $FEV_{1\%}$, PEFR, and FEV_1/PEFR in the four groups; type I, AA, AA with type I, and AA with NMP

Group	Timing of measurement	$FEV_{1\%}$ (%)		PEFR (%)		FEV_1/PEFR (ml/L/min)	
Type I (7 patients)	Pre	114.1±8.8	NS	72.4±17.5	P=0.0382	7.6±2.3	NS
	Post	110.5±11.0		62.0±11.8		7.6±2.3	
AA (14 patients)	Pre	106.9±8.6	NS	70.9±19.3	P=0.0154	7.3±1.9	NS
	Post	106.0±7.9		62.3±19.3		7.9±1.8	
AA with type I (14 patients)	Pre	112.5±12.9	P=0.0248	77.9±24.1	NS	6.6±1.4	NS
	Post	108.8±12.1		71.6±22.9		6.7±1.4	
AA with NMP (40 patients)	Pre	106.7±12.1	NS	79.0±18.1	P<0.0001	7.7±2.0	P=0.0303
	Post	104.7±15.0		66.1±17.4		8.2±2.2	

$FEV_{1\%}$ and PEFR were expressed as a ratio to the value expected for each patient based on gender, age, and height

Type I type I thyroplasty, *AA* arytenoid adduction, *NMP* neuromuscular pedicle flap implantation, *FEV1* % a ratio of forced expiratory volume in 1 second (FEV_1) to forced expiratory volume. The index is expressed as a ratio to the value expected for each patient based on gender, age, and height. *PEFR* peak expiratory flow rate. The index is expressed as a ratio to the value expected for each patient based on gender, age, and height, *Pre* preoperative, *Post* postoperative, *NS* not significant

Table 5.9 Means and standard deviations of pre- and postoperative measurements of $FEV_{1\%}$, PEFR, and FEV_1/PEFR in all AA patients

Group	Timing of measurement	$FEV_{1\%}$ (%)		PEFR (%)		FEV_1/PEFR (ml/L/min)	
3 AA groups combined (68 patients)	Pre	107.9 ± 11.7	NS	75.4 ± 19.6	$P < 0.0001$	7.4 ± 1.9	$P = 0.0058$
	Post	105.8 ± 13.2		66.5 ± 19.0		7.8 ± 2.1	

AA arytenoid adduction, *FEV1* % a ratio of forced expiratory volume in 1 second (FEV_1) to forced expiratory volume. The index is expressed as a ratio to the value expected for each patient based on gender, age, and height. *PEFR* peak expiratory flow rate. The index is expressed as a ratio to the value expected for each patient based on gender, age, and height. *Pre* preoperative, *Post* postoperative, *NS* not significant

References

1. Yumoto E, Sanuki T, Kumai Y. Immediate recurrent laryngeal nerve reconstruction and vocal outcome. Laryngoscope. 2006;116:1657–61.
2. Sanuki T, Yumoto E, Minoda R, Kodama N. The role of immediate recurrent laryngeal nerve reconstruction for thyroid cancer surgery. J Oncol. 2010;2010:846235.
3. Isshiki N. Phonosurgery: thyroplasty type I (medialization). In: Theory and practice. Tokyo: Springer; 1989. p. 82–104.
4. Hartl DM, Travagli JP, Leboulleux S, Baudin E, Brasnu DF, Schlumberger M. Clinical review: current concepts in the management of unilateral recurrent laryngeal nerve paralysis after thyroid surgery. J Clin Endocrinol Metab. 2005;90:3084–8.
5. Hagio Y. Investigation of the standard voice function value of the elderly. Larynx Jpn. 2004;16:111–21 (in Japanese).
6. Maronian N, Waugh P, Robinson L, Hillel A. Electromyographic findings in recurrent laryngeal nerve reinnervation. Ann Otol Rhinol Laryngol. 2003;112:314–23.
7. Crumley RL. Experiments in laryngeal reinnervation. Laryngoscope. 1982;92 Suppl 30:1–27.
8. Yumoto E, Sanuki T, Toya Y, Kodama N, Kumai Y. Nerve-muscle pedicle flap implantation combined with arytenoid adduction. Arch Otolaryngol Head Neck Surg. 2010;136:965–9.
9. Sheppert AD, Spirou GA, Berrebi AS, Garnett JD. Three-dimensional reconstruction of immunolabeled neuromuscular junctions in the human thyroarytenoid muscle. Laryngoscope. 2003;113:1973–6.
10. Isshiki N, Tanabe M, Sawada M. Arytenoid adduction for unilateral vocal cord paralysis. Arch Otolaryngol. 1978;104:555–8.
11. Hassan MM, Yumoto E, Kumai Y, Sanuki T, Kodama N. Vocal outcome after arytenoid adduction and ansa cervicalis transfer. Arch Otolaryngol Head Neck Surg. 2012;138:60–5.
12. Tucker HM. Reinnervation of the unilaterally paralyzed larynx. Ann Otol Rhinol Laryngol. 1977;86:789–94.
13. Tucker HM, Rusnov M. Laryngeal reinnervation for unilateral vocal cord paralysis: long-term results. Ann Otol Rhinol Laryngol. 1981;90:457–9.
14. Tucker HM. Combined laryngeal framework medicalization and reinnervation for unilateral vocal fold paralysis. Ann Otol Rhinol Laryngol. 1990;99:778–81.
15. Tucker HM. Combined surgical medicalization and nerve-muscle pedicle reinnervation for unilateral vocal fold paralysis: improved functional results and prevention of long-term deterioration of voice. J Voice. 1997;11:474–8.
16. Tucker HM. Long-term preservation of voice improvement following surgical medicalization and reinnervation for unilateral vocal fold paralysis. J Voice. 1999;13:251–6.

17. May M, Beery Q. Muscle-nerve pedicle laryngeal reinnervation. Laryngoscope. 1986;96:1196–200.
18. Anonsen CK, Patterson HC, Trachy RE, Gordon AM, Cummings CW. Reinnervation of skeletal muscle with a neuromuscular pedicle. Otolaryngol Head Neck Surg. 1985;93:48–57.
19. Chang SY. Studies of early laryngeal reinnervation. Laryngoscope. 1985;95:455–7.
20. Rice DH, Owens O, Burstein F, Verity A. The nerve-muscle pedicle: a visual, electromyographic, and histochemical study. Arch Otolaryngol. 1983;109:233–4.
21. Kumai Y, Ito T, Udaka N, Yumoto E. Effects of a nerve-muscle pedicle on the denervated rat thyroarytenoid muscle. Laryngoscope. 2006;116:1027–32.
22. Miyamaru S, Kumai Y, Ito T, Sanuki T, Yumoto E. Nerve-muscle pedicle implantation facilitates re-innervation of long-term denervated thyroarytenoid muscle in rats. Acta Otolaryngol. 2009;129:1486–92.
23. Chhetri DK, Berke GS. Ansa cervicalis nerve: review of the topographic anatomy and morphology. Laryngoscope. 1997;107:1366–72.
24. Munin MC, Rosen CA, Zullo T. Utility of laryngeal electromyography in predicting recovery after vocal fold paralysis. Arch Phys Med Rehabil. 2003;84:1150–3.
25. Smith LJ, Rosen CA, Niyonkuru C, Munin MC. Quantitative electromyography improves prediction in vocal fold paralysis. Laryngoscope. 2012;122:854–9.
26. Chhetri DK, Gerratt BR, Kreiman J, Berke GS. Combined arytenoid adduction and laryngeal reinnervation in the treatment of vocal fold paralysis. Laryngoscope. 1999;109:1928–36.
27. Aynehchi BB, McCoul ED, Sundaram K. Systematic review of laryngeal reinnervation techniques. Otolaryngol Head Neck Surg. 2010;143:749–59.
28. Lorenz RR, Esclamado RM, Teker AM, et al. Ansa cervicalis-to-recurrent laryngeal nerve anastomosis for unilateral vocal fold paralysis: experience of a single institution. Ann Otol Rhinol Laryngol. 2008;117:40–5.
29. Yumoto E, Samejima Y, Kumai Y, Haba K. Esophageal regurgitation as a cause of inspiratory distress after thyroplasty. Am J Otolaryngol. 2006;27:425–9.
30. Perie S, Roubeau B, Liesenfelt I, Chaigneau-Debono G, Bruel M, St Guily JL. Role of medialization in the improvement of breath control in unilateral vocal fold paralysis. Ann Otol Rhinol Laryngol. 2002;111:1026–33.
31. Tucker HM, Wanamaker J, Trott M, Hicks D. Complications of laryngeal framework surgery (phonosurgery). Laryngoscope. 1993;103:525–8.
32. Cotter CS, Avidano MA, Crary MA, Cassisi NJ, Gorham MM. Laryngeal complications after type I thyroplasty. Otolaryngol Head Neck Surg. 1995;113:671–3.
33. Abraham MT, Gonen M, Kraus DH. Complications of type I thyroplasty and arytenoids adduction. Laryngoscope. 2001;111:1322–9.
34. Lin HW, Bhattacharyya N. Incidence of perioperative airway complications in patients with previous medialization thyroplasty. Laryngoscope. 2009;119:675–8.
35. Rosen CA. Complications of phonosurgery: results of a national survey. Laryngoscope. 1998;108:1697–703.
36. Weinman EC, Maragos NE. Airway compromise in thyroplastic surgery. Laryngoscope. 2000;110:1082–5.
37. Nito T, Ushio M, Kimura M, Yamaguchi T, Tayama N. Analyses of risk factors for postoperative airway compromise following arytenoid adduction. Acta Otolaryngol. 2008;128:1342–7.
38. Narajos N, Toya Y, Kumai Y, Sanuki T, Yumoto E. Videolaryngoscopic assessment of laryngeal edema after arytenoid adduction. Laryngoscope. 2012;122:1104–8.
39. Cormier Y, Kashima H, Summer W, Menkes H. Airflow in unilateral vocal cord paralysis before and after Teflon injection. Thorax. 1978;33:57–61.
40. Janas JD, Waugh P, Swenson ER, Hillel A. Effect of thyroplasty on laryngeal airflow. Ann Otol Rhinol Laryngol. 1999;108:286–92.
41. Saarinen A, Rihkanen H, Lehikoinen-Soderlund S, Sovijarvi AR. Airway flow dynamics and voice acoustics after autologous fascia augmentation of paralyzed vocal fold. Ann Otol Rhinol Laryngol. 2000;109:563–7.

42. Schneider B, Kneussl M, Denk DM, Bigenzahn W. Aerodynamic measurements in medialization thyroplasty. Acta Otolaryngol. 2003;123:883–8.
43. Cantarella G, Fasano V, Maraschi B, Mazzola RF, Sambataro G. Airway resistance and airflow dynamics after fat injection into vocal folds. Ann Otol Rhinol Laryngol. 2006;115:810–15.
44. Yumoto E, Minoda R, Toya Y, Miyamaru S, Sanuki T. Changes in respiratory function after thyroplastic surgery. Acta Otolaryngol. 2010;130:132–7.
45. Empey DW. Assessment of upper airways obstruction. BMJ. 1972;3:503–5.
46. Rotman HH, Liss HP, Weg JG. Diagnosis of upper airway obstruction by pulmonary function testing. Chest. 1975;68:796–9.
47. Hirano M, Kurita S, Kiyokawa K, Sato K. Posterior glottis: morphological study in excised human larynges. Ann Otol Rhinol Laryngol. 1986;95:576–81.

Chapter 6
Summary and Future Perspectives

Abstract The contents of Chaps. 1, 2, 3, 4, and 5 are herein summarized, focusing on the fact that reinnervation of the thyroarytenoid (TA) muscle together with median location of the affected vocal fold is key in the recovery of the preparalysis normal voice of each patient. The nerve–muscle pedicle (NMP) method is useful for reinnervation of the TA muscle. Future efforts should address several issues: the length of time from unilateral vocal fold paralysis onset to implementation of the NMP procedure that can be expected to show positive effects of surgery, enhancement of the effects of the NMP method, prevention or minimization of synkinesis due to misdirected reinnervation, and alternative plans when the NMP method is unavailable bilaterally.

Keywords Nerve–muscle pedicle flap • Denervation period • Enhancement of reinnervation effects • Misdirected reinnervation

Unilateral vocal fold paralysis (UVFP) is characterized by various degrees of pathological motion impairment caused by a nervous system disorder and is an important clinical entity in otolaryngology. The extent of regeneration of nerve fibers after damage varies among patients. Significant misdirected regeneration occurs in some cases, while only slight synkinesis occurs in others. This variation is a major cause of the considerable inconsistencies in the vibratory patterns of the vocal folds among patients with UVFP. In patients with UVFP, negative effects on vocal fold vibration are caused by an off-midline position of the affected vocal fold, decreased stiffness and tension, reduced thickness of the vocal fold, atrophic changes of the thyroarytenoid (TA) muscle, and synkinetic movement of the vocal fold on the affected side. Conventional phonosurgery aims to correct glottal insufficiency by locating the affected vocal fold at the midline and to augment its mass. However, some patients do not recover their "normal" voice after surgery [1, 2]. Chapter 1 stressed that a normal voice can be attained by moving the immobile vocal fold to a median location and ensuring symmetrical bulk and tension of the unaffected vocal fold. Because conventional phonosurgical procedures aim to offer "static" adjustment of these features, the TA muscle does not function as the "body" of the immobile vocal fold and provides little contribution to voice production and tuning. Therefore, in addition to median location of the affected vocal fold, reacquisition of

© Springer Japan 2015
E. Yumoto, *Pathophysiology and Surgical Treatment of Unilateral Vocal Fold Paralysis*, DOI 10.1007/978-4-431-55354-0_6

TA muscle tonus by reinnervation is important to recover the patients' own preinjury voice with a dynamic mucosal wave.

Modern imaging techniques such as computed tomography, magnetic resonance imaging, and ultrasonography have advanced during the last four decades and now facilitate the establishment of the various causes of vocal fold paralysis. This has improved the surgical treatment of patients with previously inoperable life-threatening diseases. However, UVFP sometimes persists or even appears as a complication following surgery, resulting in breathy dysphonia and/or swallowing difficulties that affect patients' postoperative quality of life [3–6] despite the primary disease having been addressed. Thus, phonosurgical treatment for paralytic dysphonia is important to improve patients' quality of life after treatment of the primary disease. However, as shown in Chap. 2, conventional phonosurgery does not always help to recover the patient's own preinjury voice, although the voice quality usually improves to some extent after surgery. Static correction of the glottal configuration with respect to glottal closure and augmentation of the vocal fold is often insufficient to restore the vocal fold thickness, stiffness, and mass that are normally produced by TA muscle contraction.

Immediate reconstruction of the recurrent laryngeal nerve (RLN) at the time of tumor extirpation is reportedly effective in restoring vocal function after surgery [7–10]. However, when a patient seeks treatment for breathy dysphonia after the occurrence of UVFP, conventional static procedures are usually chosen. Although such procedures result in improvement of vocal function after surgery, they do not restore the normal preparalysis voice. In such persistent cases, especially those after neck surgeries, locating the peripheral stump of the RLN is not feasible; thus, nerve transfer and nerve interposition techniques cannot be applied to TA muscle reinnervation. Nerve–muscle pedicle (NMP) flap implantation may be a promising technique to facilitate reinnervation of a denervated muscle, even when the peripheral stump of the RLN is not located. However, since Tucker et al. [11–15] and May and Beery [16] reported improvement in patients' voices after the NMP procedure, no authors have reported favorable vocal function after this procedure. This paucity of data may be ascribed to the lack of consistent effects of the NMP method that has been reported in animal experiments. The author and his colleagues performed basic experiments using a UVFP animal model and revealed that NMP flap implantation to the denervated rat TA muscle facilitated recovery of the bulk of the muscle size and individual muscle fibers, neuromuscular junctions, and function as reflected on evoked electromyographic test results. Based on our results, the NMP technique has been refined and successfully applied clinically with excellent results [17, 18].

The author has performed refined NMP flap implantation combined with arytenoid adduction on more than 80 patients. Because of their favorable vocal outcomes, the number of patients who seek treatment for paralytic dysphonia at the author's institution is increasing. However, several issues remain to be resolved.

6.1 Duration from UVFP Onset to Implementation of NMP Procedure

As described in Chap. 3, animal experiments have revealed that the positive effects of the NMP method on TA muscle reinnervation become less evident as the time after denervation increases [19]. The experiments were undertaken using a rat model. Considering the lifespan of the rat (2.5–3.0 years), a 48-week duration of denervation in a rat might correspond to a >10-year duration in a human being. Thus, reinnervation of the denervated TA muscle may be possible even after several years of continuous UVFP. However, the possible time from UVFP onset to implementation of the NMP procedure with positive effects remains unclear. Thirty-two of the thirty-three patients described in Chap. 5 underwent surgery within 5 years after UVFP onset; the remaining patient underwent surgery 30 years after UVFP onset. As shown in Table 6.1, her vocal function at 12 and 26 months postoperatively improved compared to that at 6 months after surgery, although the final vocal function parameters did not reach their normal ranges. The poor pulmonary function of this patient may have been a cause of these results. As a whole, all voice parameters at all postoperative visits (1, 3, 6, 12, and 24 months) improved significantly compared with their preoperative values. Moreover, the measurements of all voice parameters excluding jitter, shimmer, and pitch range were within their respective reference ranges at 24 months after surgery. Further accumulation of a larger number of patients with varying durations of UVFP is necessary to investigate this issue further.

6.2 Enhancement of the Effects of the NMP Method

The presence of muscle fibers is a prerequisite for successful reinnervation. In addition, because acetylcholine receptors (AchRs) are the target for regenerating axon sprouts during the reinnervation process, the muscle fibers should retain AchRs to

Table 6.1 Vocal function of a patient who had NMP procedure combined with arytenoid adduction 366 months after UVFP onset

Period after surgery (months)	MPT (s)	MFR (mL/s)	Jitter (%)	Shimmer (%)	HNR (dB)	G	B	Pitch range (semitone)
Preop	3.5	266	4.472	9.022	5.376	1.0	1.0	8
1	6.5	231	4.72	20.436	2.475	1.7	1.0	12
3	5.8	231	5.026	8.862	6.3	1.7	0.7	12
6	7.5	182	6.806	15.421	3.585	1.0	0.7	15
12	11.3	209	1.767	5.053	8.268	0.7	0.3	11
26	10.7	184	1.528	5.359	8.996	1.0	1.0	13

MPT maximum phonation time, *MFR* mean airflow rate, *HNR* harmonics-to-noise ratio
G grade overall, *B* breathiness

accommodate the new connections. In theory, a higher number of preserved AchRs leads to more efficient reinnervation. Therefore, prevention of both TA muscle atrophy and AchR disappearance may enhance the effects of the NMP method. Prevention of motor neuron apoptosis in the nucleus ambiguus (NA) is also important, especially when nerve injury occurs close to the NA. For example, administration of basic fibroblast growth factor (bFGF) at the injured site has been shown to facilitate regeneration of motor fibers after RLN injury [20]. Furthermore, endogenous bFGF may contribute to the prevention of neuronal death induced by peripheral RLN injury [21, 22]. Additionally, gene therapy involving the transfer of genes for neurotrophic factors such as IGF-1 and GDNF into denervated laryngeal muscles or into the nucleus ambiguus may be a promising approach for the prevention of atrophic changes of the denervated TA muscle [23]. However, gene therapies have certain safety, ethical, and cost issues related to clinical application.

Another possible strategy is to accelerate regeneration of sprouting nerve fibers [24, 25]. The growth cone plays an important role in guiding axon regeneration. Silver et al. revealed that the L-type voltage-operated calcium channel (VOCC) exists in all regions of the growth cone, usually at the base of processes extending from the growth cone palm [26]. The author and his colleagues reported that nimodipine, an L-type VOCC antagonist, promoted reinnervation of denervated rat TA muscles following NMP flap implantation [27]. Nimodipine also expedited the effects of the NMP method on long-term denervated TA muscles [28]. Although nimodipine is not currently approved by the Japanese Ministry of Health, Labor and Welfare, it has been used clinically in the United States and Europe to treat hypertension and prevent vasospasm after subarachnoid hemorrhage. Translational research may be required to clinically apply L-type VOCC antagonists for this novel indication.

6.3 Synkinesis Due to Misdirected Reinnervation

The author classified glottal configuration in patients with UVFP into three types (see Chap. 4). In type A glottal configuration, the thickness of the affected vocal fold during phonation was equal to or slightly thinner than that of the healthy vocal fold. The affected fold during phonation in this type is directed medially, not superomedially. Only a slight glottal gap was present between the vocal processes during phonation. Patients whose affected fold was thinner than its mate during phonation were further classified into types B and C. In type B glottal configuration, the affected fold remained thin during both phonation and inhalation. Type C was characterized by one or two paradoxical movements of the affected fold that were directed medially, not superomedially, during inhalation. The affected fold in type B was directed superomedially and that in type C was hardly recognizable on the coronal image during phonation. There was a prominent glottal gap between the vocal processes during phonation in type B and C glottal configurations. Of the 37 patients examined in Sect. 4.3.2, 15 (40.5 %) were classified as type C. Although reinnervation occurred in patients with type C glottal configuration, their vocal function did not improve because of misdirected reinnervation. In contrast, the vocal function in patients with type A glottal configuration was significantly more favorable than that in patients with type C [29]. Because of the random distribution between the adductor and abductor nerve fibers within the RLN or vagal nerve bundle, no methods are at present available to prevent or minimize misdirected reinnervation after the occurrence of severe nerve injury (grade III, IV, or V according to the Sunderland classification [30]).

6.4 Unavailability of NMP Flap Formation

A significant number of patients with UVFP have a history of neck operations, mainly thyroid and esophageal cancer extirpation accompanied by varying degrees of neck dissection. In such cases, the ACN and sternohyoid (SH) muscle may have been resected and not be available for reinnervation of the TA muscle. When an NMP flap cannot be harvested on the affected side, one alternative is to create an NMP flap on the other side and implant the flap over the midline. Actually, an NMP flap was harvested on the unaffected side in two of the nine patients after completion of their thyroid cancer operations in the series described in Sect. 5.4 (Table 5.3). Additionally, in the remaining seven patients (and in two patients after esophageal cancer operations), an NMP flap was made on the affected side after electrostimulation results confirmed the presence of a functional ACN. During the same period as in the series in Sect. 5.4, an NMP flap could not be created in ten patients (four with thyroid cancer and six with esophageal cancer). As shown in Fig. 5.2, when the ACN and SH muscle are not available for reinnervation, arytenoid adduction (AA) alone or AA combined with a medialization procedure is performed despite the fact that no TA muscle reinnervation occurs. Paniello anastomosed the hypoglossal nerve with the peripheral stump of the RLN in nine patients and reported excellent voice quality, resolution of preoperative aspiration, and minimal morbidity due to deficiency of hypoglossal nerve function [31]. However, his method required a $\geq$3-cm length of the peripheral RLN stump, which is not feasible in UVFP patients after neck surgery. Therefore, no practical method for reinnervation of the TA muscle exists when the NMP flap cannot be harvested bilaterally.

References

1. Kimura M, Nito T, Imagawa H, Tayama N, Chan RW. Collagen injection as a supplement to arytenoid adduction for vocal fold paralysis. Ann Otol Rhinol Laryngol. 2008;117:430–6.
2. Mortensen M, Carroll L, Woo P. Arytenoid adduction with medialization laryngoplasty versus injection or medialization laryngoplasty: the role of the arytenoidopexy. Laryngoscope. 2009;119:827–31.
3. Smith E, Taylor M, Mendoza M, Barkmeier J, Lemke J, Hoffman H. Spasmodic dysphonia and vocal fold paralysis: outcomes of voice problems on work-related functioning. J Voice. 1998;12:223–32.

4. Benninger MS, Ahuja AS, Gardner G, Grywalski C. Assessing outcomes for dysphonic patients. J Voice. 1998;12:540–50.
5. Baba M, Natsugoe S, Shimada M, Nakano S, Noguchi Y, Kawachi K, Kusano C, Aikou T. Does hoarseness of voice from recurrent nerve paralysis after esophagectomy for carcinoma influence patient quality of life? J Am Coll Surg. 1999;188:231–6.
6. Fang TJ, Li HY, Glicklich RE, Chen YH, Wang PC, Chuang HF. Quality of life measures and predictors for adults with unilateral vocal cord paralysis. Laryngoscope. 2008;118:1837–41.
7. Miyauchi A, Matsusaka K, Kihara M, Matsuzuka F, Hirai K, Yokozawa T, Kobayashi A, Kuma K. The role of ansa-to-recurrent laryngeal nerve anastomosis in operations for thyroid cancer. Eur J Surg. 1998;164:927–33.
8. Miyauchi A, Inoue H, Tomoda C, Fukushima M, Kihara M, Higashiyama T, Takamura Y, Ito Y, Kobayashi K, Miya A. Improvement in phonation after reconstruction of the recurrent laryngeal nerve in patients with thyroid cancer invading the nerve. Surgery. 2009;146:1056–62.
9. Yumoto E, Sanuki T, Kumai Y. Immediate recurrent laryngeal nerve reconstruction and vocal outcome. Laryngoscope. 2006;116:1657–61.
10. Sanuki T, Yumoto E, Minoda R, Kodama N. The role of immediate recurrent laryngeal nerve reconstruction for thyroid cancer surgery. J Oncol. 2010;846235.
11. Tucker HM. Reinnervation of the unilaterally paralyzed larynx. Ann Otol Rhinol Laryngol. 1977;86:789–94.
12. Tucker HM, Rusnov M. Laryngeal reinnervation for unilateral vocal cord paralysis: long-term results. Ann Otol Rhinol Laryngol. 1981;90:457–9.
13. Tucker HM. Combined laryngeal framework medicalization and reinnervation for unilateral vocal fold paralysis. Ann Otol Rhinol Laryngol. 1990;99:778–81.
14. Tucker HM. Combined surgical medicalization and nerve-muscle pedicle reinnervation for unilateral vocal fold paralysis: improved functional results and prevention of long-term deterioration of voice. J Voice. 1997;11:474–8.
15. Tucker HM. Long-term preservation of voice improvement following surgical medicalization and reinnervation for unilateral vocal fold paralysis. J Voice. 1999;13:251–6.
16. May M, Beery Q. Muscle-nerve pedicle laryngeal reinnervation. Laryngoscope. 1986;96:1196–200.
17. Yumoto E, Sanuki T, Toya Y, Kodama N, Kumai Y. Nerve-muscle pedicle flap implantation combined with arytenoid adduction. Arch Otolaryngol Head Neck Surg. 2010;136:965–9.
18. Hassan MM, Yumoto E, Baraka A, Sanuki T, Kodama N. Arytenoid rotation and nerve-muscle pedicle transfer in paralytic dysphonia. Laryngoscope. 2011;121:1018–22.
19. Miyamaru S, Kumai Y, Ito T, Sanuki T, Yumoto E. Nerve-muscle pedicle implantation facilitates re-innervation of long-term denervated thyroarytenoid muscle in rats. Acta Otolaryngol. 2009;129:1486–92.
20. Komori M. Effects of neurotrophic factors on regeneration of denervated recurrent laryngeal nerve in the rat. Pract Otorhinolaryngol. 1999;92:677–86. (in Japanese)
21. Sanuki T, Yumoto E, Komori M, Hyodo M. Expression of fibroblast growth factor-2 in the nucleus ambiguus following recurrent laryngeal nerve injury in the rat. Laryngoscope. 2000;110:2128–34.
22. Huber K, Meisinger C, Grotiie C. Expression of fibroblast growth factor-2 in hypoglossal motoneurons is stimulated by peripheral nerve injury. J Comp Neurol. 1997;382:189–98.
23. Shiotani A, Saito K, Araki K, Moro K, Watabe K. Gene therapy for laryngeal paralysis. Ann Otol Rhinol Laryngol. 2007;116:115–22.
24. Hydman J, Remahl S, Bjorck G, Svensson M, Mattsson P. Nimodipine improves reinnervation and neuromuscular function after injury to the recurrent laryngeal nerve in the rat. Ann Otol Rhinol Laryngol. 2007;116:623–30.
25. Hydman J, Mattsson P. Preserved regeneration and functional recovery of the injured recurrent laryngeal nerve after secondary surgical repair in adult rats. Ann Otol Rhinol Laryngol. 2009;118:73–80.

26. Silver RA, Lamb AG, Bolsover SR. Calcium hotspots caused by L-channel clustering promote morphological changes in neuronal growth cones. Nature. 1990;343:751–4.
27. Nishimoto K, Kumai Y, Minoda R, Yumoto E. Nimodipine accelerates re-innervation of denervated rat thyroarytenoid muscle following nerve-muscle pedicle implantation. Laryngoscope. 2012;122:606–13.
28. Nishimoto K, Kumai Y, Sanuki T, Minoda R, Yumoto E. The impact of nimodipine administration combined with nerve-muscle pedicle implantation on long-term denervated rat thyroarytenoid muscle. Laryngoscope. 2013;123:952–9.
29. Yumoto E, Sanuki T, Minoda R, Kumai Y, Nishimoto K. Glottal configuration in unilaterally paralyzed larynx and vocal function. Acta Otolaryngol. 2013;133:187–93.
30. Sunderland S. A classification of peripheral nerve injuries producing loss of function. Brain. 1951;74:491–516.
31. Paniello RC. Laryngeal reinnervation with the hypoglossal nerve: II. Clinical evaluation and early patient experience. Laryngoscope. 2000;110:739–48.